Natural Infection Fighters

Effective Herbal Antibiotics for Everyday Use

Jessica Brown

© Copyright 2024 - All rights reserved.

The content contained within this book may not be reproduced, duplicated or transmitted without direct written permission from the author or the publisher. Under no circumstances will any blame or legal responsibility be

held against
the publisher, or author, for any damages, reparation, or monetary loss due to the information contained within this book, either directly or indirectly.

Legal Notice:

This book is copyright protected. It is only for personal use. You cannot amend, distribute, sell, use, quote or paraphrase any part, or the content within this book, without the consent of the author or publisher.

Disclaimer Notice:

Please note the information contained within this document is for educational and entertainment purposes only. All effort has been executed to present accurate, up to date, reliable, complete information. No warranties of any kind are declared or implied. Readers acknowledge that the author is not engaging in the rendering of legal, financial, medical or professional advice. The content within this book has been derived from various sources. Please consult a licensed professional before attempting any techniques outlined in this book.

By reading this document, the reader agrees that under no circumstances is the author responsible for any losses, direct or indirect, that are incurred as a result of the use of information contained within this document, including, but not limited to, errors, omissions, or inaccuracies.

Table of Contents

INTRODUCTION 7
CHAPTER I: The Science Behind Herbal Antibiotics 9
Understanding Infections and Immunity 9
Types of infections (bacterial, viral, fungal, etc.) 11
How the immune system works 13
Mechanisms of Herbal Antibiotics 14
How herbs combat pathogens 16
Comparison with conventional antibiotics 18
Scientific Studies and Evidence 20
CHAPTER II: Getting Started with Herbal Remedies 23
Basic Principles of Herbal Medicine 23
Herbal preparation methods (tinctures, teas, capsules, etc.) 25
Dosage and administration 28
Safety and Precautions 30
Potential side effects and interactions 32
Guidelines for safe use 34
CHAPTER III: Top 10 Herbal Antibiotics........................... 36
Garlic (Allium sativum) 36
Echinacea (Echinacea spp.) 38
Goldenseal (Hydrastis canadensis) 40

Ginger (Zingiber officinale) 42

Turmeric (Curcuma longa).. 44

Oregano (Origanum vulgare) Properties, uses, and preparations 46

CHAPTER IV : Herbal Antibiotics for Common Ailments .. 49

Colds, flu, bronchitis 49

Cuts, burns, acne 51

Food poisoning, stomach flu 53

Urinary Tract Infections 56

CHAPTER V: Creating Your Herbal Medicine Cabinet 59

Essential Herbs to Keep on Hand Detailed list and descriptions 59

Tools and Supplies Needed Equipment for preparation and storage 62

Recipes for Herbal Remedies Step-by-step guides for common preparations 65

CHAPTER VI: Integrating Herbal Antibiotics into Daily Life 68

Preventative Use of Herbs 68

Strengthening the immune system 70

Travel kit essentials 72

Tips for staying healthy on the go 73

Combining Herbs with Modern Medicine 76

How to work with healthcare providers 77

CHAPTER VII: Advanced Topics in Herbal Antibiotics 80

Herbal Synergies and Combinations 80

Combining herbs for enhanced effect 82

Recipes and formulations 84

Cultivating Your Own Medicinal Herbs 86

Gardening tips and techniques 87

Best herbs to grow at home 89

CHAPTER VIII: Herbal Antibiotics for Children and Pets . 92

Special Considerations for Children 92

Dosage adjustments 94

Safe herbs for children 96

Herbal Remedies for Pets 98

Common ailments and treatments 100

Guidelines for safe use 102

CHAPTER IX: Troubleshooting and Overcoming Challenges 105

Common Problems and Solutions 105

Addressing non-responsiveness to herbs 107

Managing side effects 109

Building a Support System 111

Finding reliable information and support 113

Joining herbal communities 115

CHAPTER X : Case Studies and Success Stories 118
Real-Life Examples... 118
Detailed case studies 122
Key takeaways and insights 126
CONCLUSION **129**

INTRODUCTION

Greetings and welcome to Natural Infection Fighters: Natural Antibiotics That Work Well for Everyday Use. For people looking for holistic health treatments, the growing popularity of natural therapies presents a hopeful option in a world where synthetic antibiotics are used more and more. Combining cutting-edge scientific research with age-old knowledge, this e-book aims to lead you through the intriguing and productive field of herbal antibiotic research.

Many civilizations have used herbal medicines for millennia to cure infections and advance health. In contrast to their synthetic equivalents, which may cause side effects and antibiotic resistance, natural antibiotics function in tandem with the body, frequently offering a more delicate yet efficient healing method. This e-book aims to illuminate the advantages of these natural therapies by emphasizing their effectiveness, safety, and suitability for regular use.

There are many different herbs that you may get that have antiviral, antibacterial, and antifungal qualities. This book covers a wide range of simple natural remedies to include daily, from well-known herbs like olive leaf and goldenseal to lesser-known yet potent ones like garlic and ginger.

Starting from the beginning, we will examine the science underlying herbal antibiotics and comprehend how they work to treat illnesses. You'll discover safe preparation and usage methods for these herbs and helpful guidance on where to find, store, and use them. Every chapter explores a particular illness and offers thorough herbal remedies for prevalent infections, giving you the information to address health problems safely and efficiently.

By the time you finish reading this e-book, you will have a thorough grasp of herbal antibiotics, the ability to make wise decisions regarding your health, and the motivation to use these all-natural therapies in your daily routine. Join us on this adventure to learn about the natural anti-infection agents that can revolutionize your view of health and recovery.

CHAPTER I

The Science Behind Herbal Antibiotics

Understanding Infections and Immunity

Pathogens, including bacteria, viruses, fungi, and parasites, cause infections. These microscopic intruders can cause everything from a cold to tuberculosis or HIV/AIDS. Maintaining health and creating effective therapies requires understanding how these viruses work and how our bodies respond.

Bacterial infections are prevalent and can affect any bodily area. Single-celled bacteria may survive in many situations. Pathogenic bacteria can cause serious illnesses, although many helpful bacteria aid digestion. Strep throat, UTIs, and pneumonia are common bacterial infections. Pathogen poisons harm tissues and cause inflammation, the body's response to injury and illness. Alternative treatments for bacterial infections, such as herbal medicines, are needed due to antibiotic-resistant bacteria.

Virus-caused illnesses provide unique challenges.

Smaller than bacteria, viruses multiply in host cells. Viruses exploit cellular machinery within the body to make additional viruses, often killing host cells. This can cause influenza, HIV, and COVID-19. Viral infections are rarely treated with antibiotics. Antivirals and vaccines are the main treatments for viral illnesses. However, they have limits. The immune system uses specialized cells to recognize and destroy viral infections.

Fungal infections, albeit rare, can create serious health issues. Fungal infections can affect the skin, nails, lungs, and other organs. Fungal infections include athlete's foot, yeast, and histoplasmosis. Due to immune system weakness or flora imbalance, these illnesses often arise. Antifungal drugs address these illnesses, but like bacteria and viruses, fungi can acquire resistance, making treatment more challenging.

Parasites live on or inside hosts and get their nourishment from them. Protozoa, helminths, and ectoparasites like lice and ticks can cause parasitic infections. Plasmodium protozoa and parasitic worms, which cause malaria and schistosomiasis, are major health issues in tropical climates. Antiparasitic medicines and supportive care are often needed for these illnesses.

Our immune system is sophisticated enough to fight these many infections. It uses organs, tissues, and cells to detect and remove external intruders. The two primary levels are innate and adaptive immunity. Pathogens are promptly fought by innate immunity.

Physical barriers like skin and mucous membranes inhibit germs. The innate immune system uses macrophages, neutrophils, and natural killer cells to eliminate infections that pass these barriers. These cells use pattern recognition receptors to identify infections and launch inflammatory reactions to destroy them.

However, adaptive immunity is more specific and activates more slowly. B and T lymphocytes identify pathogen antigens. In response to pathogens, B cells can create antibodies that neutralize or destroy them. T cells can kill infected cells or coordinate immune responses. Memory is crucial to adaptive immunity. The immune system remembers a pathogen, allowing it to respond sooner and more effectively if it is met again. This approach makes vaccines effective by training the immune system to recognize and fight infections.

The immune-infection relationship is complicated and dynamic. Pathogens can mutate quickly, hide in host cells, or dampen immunological responses to avoid the immune system. As dangers evolve, the immune system adjusts to fight them. Understanding this delicate balance is crucial to creating novel medicines and preventive measures to combat infectious diseases.

Types of infections (bacterial, viral, fungal, etc.)

Infections from bacteria, viruses, fungi, and parasites are serious health issues. Pathogens behave differently and require different preventative and treatment methods. Understanding infection types is essential for managing and fighting diseases.

Bacterial infections are caused by single-celled germs that may survive in many conditions. Many bacteria are benign and help digestion and nutrition cycling. However, pathogenic bacteria can cause significant infections. Common bacterial infections include strep throat, urinary tract infections, and bacterial pneumonia, usually caused by Streptococcus pneumoniae. Due to microbial toxins, these infections can induce fever, inflammation, and pain. Antibiotics are the primary therapy for bacterial infections, although antibiotic-resistant forms like MRSA have made alternative therapies and preventive measures necessary.

Virus-caused infections are complicated. Smaller than bacteria, viruses multiply in host cells. They inject genetic material into host cells to hijack their machinery and make new viruses, often killing the cell. The SARS-CoV-2 pandemic, the common cold, influenza, HIV/AIDS, and COVID-19 are viral illnesses. Unlike bacteria, viruses cannot be treated with antibiotics. Antivirals and vaccinations, which train the immune system to fight viruses, are used instead. However, viruses' tremendous mutation rate can create new strains that resist therapies and vaccines.

Fungi—yeasts, molds, and mushrooms—cause fungal infections. Fungal infections can harm skin, nails, lungs, and other organs. Athletic foot, caused by dermatophytes; yeast infections, caused by Candida species; and histoplasmosis, which can affect the lungs and other organs, are common fungal illnesses. These infections usually result from immune system weakness or microbial imbalance. Fungi, like bacteria and viruses, can acquire resistance to antifungals, making treatment more challenging.

Parasites reside on or inside hosts and steal nutrition, causing parasitic diseases. Protozoa, helminths, and ectoparasites like lice and ticks can cause parasitic infections. Plasmodium protozoa-caused malaria remains a severe health issue in many tropical regions. For instance, Giardia lamblia causes giardiasis, whereas parasitic worms produce schistosomiasis. Antiparasitic medicines and supportive care are often needed for these illnesses.

These typical categories are joined by mixed infections, which involve many pathogens, and nosocomial infections, which are spread in hospitals. Mixed infections can be challenging to diagnose and treat because germs require various treatments. Hospitals have highly resistant bacteria, making nosocomial infections severe and difficult to cure.

The variations between these infections must be understood for accurate diagnosis, treatment, and prevention. Medical experts must consider how each pathogen affects the body while establishing infectious disease strategies. By learning more about these viruses and how they cause disease, we may enhance public health and develop more effective medicines to combat these changing dangers.

How the immune system works

The immune system is a complex network of cells, tissues, and organs that fights bacteria, viruses, fungi, and parasites. Its main job is to recognize and remove foreign invaders while separating them from healthy cells. The immune system uses innate and adaptive immunity to keep you healthy and avoid illnesses.

First-line defense, innate immunity, respond swiftly to infections. This immunity targets broad microbial traits rather than individual diseases. Skin and mucous membranes prevent infections from entering the body, forming innate immunity. The innate immune system uses macrophages, neutrophils, and natural killer cells to eliminate invaders if these barriers are overcome. Pattern recognition receptors on these cells identify pathogens' molecular patterns. These cells launch an inflammatory response following discovery to contain and remove the pathogen. Inflammation increases blood flow to the infection site, delivering immune cells and encouraging recovery.

Acquired or adaptive immunity is more specialized and takes longer to activate than innate immunity. It involves B and T lymphocytes that identify pathogen antigens. B cells develop into plasma cells that generate antibodies when pathogens are recognized. These antibodies mark pathogens for immune cell destruction or neutralization by binding to their surface antigens. Helper and cytotoxic T cells are the major types of T cells. Cytotoxic T cells destroy infected cells by adhering to their surface antigens, whereas helper T cells release cytokines to signal other immune cells to respond.

Memory is crucial to adaptive immunity. After exposure to a disease, the immune system generates memory cells that remember its antigens. This allows a faster and more efficient response to further pathogen exposure. This is why vaccines work: they introduce innocuous pathogen components to train the immune system to recognize and fight them without causing disease.

The immune system contains organs and tissues that help immune cells grow and operate. Primary lymphoid organs like the bone marrow and thymus create and develop immune cells. The thymus matures T cells, while the bone marrow makes all blood cells, including immune cells. Lymph nodes, spleen, and tonsils coordinate immune responses. Pathogens are trapped in lymph nodes, allowing immune cells to respond. Spleens filter blood, remove old or damaged cells and germs, and aid immunological responses.

The immune system is highly integrated and active, protecting the body from infections and disorders. Its ability to identify self from non-self, recognize many diseases and recall earlier interactions makes it a potent protection mechanism. Immune system malfunctions can cause autoimmune diseases, where the body attacks its cells, or immunodeficiency disorders, which impair infection defense. Developing innovative therapies and vaccinations, enhancing public health, and controlling immune-related disorders requires understanding the immune system.

Mechanisms of Herbal Antibiotics

Traditional medicine has used herbal antibiotics to treat infections and promote health for ages. Plant-based medicines have antibacterial characteristics that target bacteria, viruses, fungi, and parasites. Herbal antibiotics combine plant chemicals to fight infections.

One of the main effects of herbal antibiotics is the breakdown of bacterial cell walls. Many antibacterial plants contain flavonoids, tannins, and essential oils that disrupt bacterial cell wall formation, causing cell lysis and death. For instance, garlic (Allium sativum) contains allicin, which disrupts bacterial cell membranes, making it robust against many germs. Oregano (Origanum vulgare) essential oil contains carvacrol and thymol, which weaken bacterial cell walls and limit growth.

Herbal antibiotics limit microbial protein synthesis. Several plants include chemicals that bind to bacterial ribosomes, inhibiting crucial protein synthesis. This prevents bacteria growth and reproduction. Goldenseal (Hydrastis canadensis) contains berberine, an alkaloid that inhibits pathogenic bacterium protein production.

Herbal antibiotics can also inhibit pathogen reproduction and survival by inhibiting nucleic acid synthesis. Certain plant chemicals hinder DNA and RNA synthesis enzymes, reducing bacterial and viral multiplication. Neem (Azadirachta indica) contains chemicals that inhibit bacteria and viral nucleic acid production, decreasing their capacity to increase and infect.

Herbal antibiotics alter the immune system to boost defenses. Immunomodulatory herbs boost macrophages, natural killer cells, and lymphocytes. Echinacea (Echinacea spp.) boosts the immune system by increasing white blood cell production and infection resistance. Herbal antibiotics work well because they directly fight germs and boost immunity.

Many natural antibiotics also work through antioxidants. ROS buildup causes oxidative stress, which damages microbial cells. Many plants contain antioxidants, including polyphenols and vitamins that neutralize ROS and boost antibacterial activity. Curcumin, the main chemical in turmeric (Curcuma longa), has antioxidant capabilities that destroy pathogen cellular components and impede growth.

Anti-inflammatory effects of herbal antibiotics minimize infection-related inflammation. The immune system responds to infection with inflammation, but excessive inflammation can harm tissue and aggravate symptoms. Ginger (Zingiber officinale) contains anti-inflammatory gingerols that relieve symptoms and fight disease.

Due to their complexity and variety of components, herbal antibiotics prevent resistance, unlike synthetic antibiotics. Herbal antibiotics target numerous areas of microbe physiology, making them less likely to acquire resistance. This multi-target approach hinders pathogen adaptation and survival.

Herbal antibiotics damage microbial cell walls, impede protein and nucleic acid synthesis, modulate the immune system, and have antioxidant and anti-inflammatory actions. These methods directly attack germs and boost the body's natural defenses, making herbal medicines useful in infection prevention. Understanding these pathways can help design more effective and sustainable infectious illness treatments.

How herbs combat pathogens

For millennia, herbs have treated infections and other diseases. Their complicated chemical compositions disturb the life cycles and biological activities of bacteria, viruses, fungi, and parasites. Herbs' versatility makes them powerful friends in fighting viral diseases.

Herbs fight infections by destroying cell walls and membranes. Many herbs contain essential oils, flavonoids, and tannins that can harm microbial cell walls. This disturbance damages the cell wall or membrane, causing lysis and death. The vital oils of oregano and thyme contain carvacrol and thymol. These chemicals increase bacterial membrane permeability and spill critical cellular contents, killing the bacteria.

Protein synthesis inhibition is also essential. Some herbs include chemicals that disrupt microbial ribosomes, which translate genetic information into proteins. Pathogens cannot grow, reproduce, or operate without these proteins. Berberine, an alkaloid in goldenseal, binds to the bacterial ribosome and prevents protein synthesis, reducing bacterial life. This inhibits bacterial growth and reproduction, eliminating illnesses.

Herbs hinder nucleic acid synthesis to kill infections.

Herbal chemicals can block DNA and RNA synthesis enzymes, preventing pathogen replication. Neem, a popular traditional medicine plant, contains chemicals that inhibit bacterium and viral DNA reproduction, decreasing their spread. Herbal remedies prevent infection by suppressing these vital processes.

Immunomodulatory herbs boost the body's defenses. They boost macrophage, natural killer, and lymphocyte activity, helping the body fight infections. Echinacea is a popular immunostimulant. Increasing white blood cell formation and activity increases the immunological response and pathogen detection.

Antioxidant-rich herbs fight pathogen oxidative stress.

ROS destroys cells, causing oxidative stress. Many plants contain antioxidants, such as polyphenols, flavonoids, and vitamins, that neutralize ROS, damaging pathogen cells. Curcumin, the main ingredient in turmeric, contains antioxidant characteristics that impair microbe biological activities, making it difficult to survive and multiply.

Many herbs' anti-inflammatory characteristics assist in regulating infection symptoms and speed healing. Infection causes inflammation, but severe inflammation can harm tissue and aggravate symptoms. Ginger and turmeric relieve symptoms and fight infection using antimicrobial substances. Gingerol reduces inflammation and is antibacterial, making it beneficial against many diseases.

Herbs' capacity to attack several targets concurrently is vital to pathogen fight. Unlike manufactured antibiotics, herbs include many chemicals that affect a pathogen's biology. Complexity makes pathogen resistance harder. Pathogens must evolve resistance mechanisms to counter herbal medicines' multidimensional attack, which is statistically less plausible than single-agent antibiotic resistance.

In summary, herbs fight infections by breaking cell walls and membranes, limiting protein and nucleic acid synthesis, boosting immunity, giving antioxidants, and lowering inflammation. Their diverse chemical compositions allow them to assault germs on several fronts, making them practical and sustainable infection treatments. Understanding these mechanisms shows herbal therapy's promise in traditional and modern medicine.

Comparison with conventional antibiotics

Traditional and herbal antibiotics are two strategies in the battle against infections, each with pros and cons. Herbal antibiotics, made from plants, provide a centuries-old alternative to highly potent and commonly used conventional antibiotics, resulting from modern pharmacology. When these two methods are compared, disparities in their overall efficacy, side effects, and mechanisms of action become apparent.

Most conventional antibiotics are either artificially or obtained from microorganisms like fungi and bacteria. These antibiotics are made to target specific bacterial processes or structures specifically. Tetracyclines, for example, block protein synthesis by attaching to bacterial ribosomes, whereas penicillins interfere with forming bacterial cell walls. Conventional antibiotics are an excellent treatment option for bacterial infections because of their specificity, which can result in quick and efficient bacterial eradication. Their focused activity, meanwhile, may also hurt the emergence of antibiotic resistance. Bacteria can rapidly adjust to these methods by gaining resistance genes from other bacteria or genetically changing their DNA to become resistant.

On the other hand, herbal antibiotics are made of intricate blends of organic substances present in plants. These substances frequently target several pathways at once to act in concert to provide antibacterial effects. Garlic, for instance, has chemicals called allicin that break down bacterial cell membranes. Other garlic components may strengthen the immune system or prevent the formation of new proteins. Unlike traditional antibiotics, this multimodal strategy hinders the development of bacterial resistance. Pathogens would have to simultaneously evolve several resistance mechanisms due to the complexity of herbal antibiotics. This is less plausible than developing resistance to a conventional antibiotic that targets a single target.

An additional significant divergence can be found in the adverse reaction profiles of conventional and natural antibiotics. From minor gastrointestinal discomfort to severe allergic responses and antibiotic-associated diarrhea, conventional antibiotics can have a broad spectrum of adverse effects. They may also throw off the delicate balance of good bacteria in the digestive system, resulting in secondary illnesses like colitis caused by Clostridium difficile. Contrarily, herbal antibiotics are typically thought to be kinder to the body and to have fewer, milder side effects. This is partially because they are frequently utilized in their entirety or as extracts that have a combination of supporting and active ingredients that can lessen negative impacts.

Herbal medicines can, however, vary more in their effectiveness and uniformity than synthetic antibiotics. Antibiotics used in pharmaceuticals are produced by strict guidelines, guaranteeing constant potency and purity. The quantities of the active ingredients in herbal antibiotics can vary greatly depending on several factors, including the type of plant, growth environment, and extraction technique. This unpredictability may reduce their efficacy and complicate dosing. Furthermore, even though the use of herbal antibiotics is supported by a significant body of traditional knowledge and some scientific studies, these treatments have typically received less clinical trial research than conventional antibiotics, which undergo extensive testing to ensure their safety and effectiveness.

Herbal antibiotics frequently have an advantage in terms of sustainability and accessibility. A variety of locally cultivated and sustainably collected medicinal plants can provide an inexpensive and easily accessible source of antimicrobial treatment, particularly in areas with limited access to traditional healthcare. Although they are widely accessible worldwide, conventional antibiotics can be costly and necessitate complex manufacturing procedures.

In conclusion, each type of antibiotic—herbal and conventional—has advantages and disadvantages of its own. While they provide effective, focused treatment choices, conventional antibiotics also carry a higher risk of resistance and adverse consequences. Although they have fewer side effects and a reduced risk of resistance, herbal antibiotics offer a more comprehensive, multi-targeted approach. However, standardization and clinical validation of these drugs present problems. By being aware of these distinctions, physicians can treat infections with more knowledge. They may even combine the use of both classes of antibiotics to improve patient outcomes and fight antibiotic resistance.

Scientific Studies and Evidence

Scientific studies and evidence underpin our understanding and validation of conventional and alternative treatments, including herbal antibiotics. In recent decades, scientific study on natural antibiotics has grown in popularity. The necessity for antibiotic alternatives, mainly due to drug resistance, drives this interest. Laboratory investigations, clinical trials, and meta-analyses help researchers comprehend herbal antibiotics' benefits and drawbacks.

Laboratory tests, the first step in scientific research, have shown that herbs have antimicrobial properties. Herbal extracts are evaluated against bacteria, viruses, and fungi in vitro. Garlic (Allium sativum) has been shown to have antibacterial properties against many infections, including MRSA. This impact is caused by allicin, which disrupts bacterial cell membranes and metabolism. Oregano oil, high in carvacrol and thymol, inhibits several bacterial species, validating its historical usage as an antibacterial.

Animal experiments support herbal antibiotic efficacy beyond in vitro research. These studies explain herbal chemical pharmacokinetics and adverse effects in live organisms. In rat models, berberine, an alkaloid in goldenseal, inhibits bacterial growth and alters the immune response, improving infection resistance. Such investigations are essential for evaluating doses and toxicities before human trials.

Human clinical trials are the gold standard for therapeutic safety and efficacy. Herbal antibiotics have fewer clinical trials than conventional medications, but the outcomes are promising. In a randomized controlled trial of echinacea extract for upper respiratory infections, participants who received the herb had significantly fewer symptoms than those who received a placebo. Cranberry extract reduced urinary tract infection rates in another clinical investigation, suggesting its efficacy as a prophylactic strategy.

To assess herbal antibiotic efficacy, systematic reviews and meta-analyses combine data from several studies. These studies reveal trends, effectiveness, and research gaps. According to a meta-analysis, tea tree oil is beneficial against a variety of bacteria and fungi, especially in treating skin infections. Healthcare providers seeking evidence-based antibiotic alternatives benefit from such detailed reviews.

Despite promising results, herbal antibiotics need more rigorous, high-quality research to prove their efficacy and safety. Many studies have tiny sample sizes, unstandardized herbal formulations, and different methodologies. To scientifically validate herbal antibiotics, well-designed clinical trials and established methodologies must address these difficulties.

Finally, scientific studies and data are essential for comprehending herbal antibiotics' potential. Laboratory studies, animal research, clinical trials, and meta-analyses support herbal antibiotics for diverse infections. Research and thorough scientific confirmation are needed to integrate these natural therapies into mainstream healthcare to supplement conventional antibiotics and combat antibiotic resistance.

CHAPTER II

Getting Started with Herbal Remedies

Basic Principles of Herbal Medicine

Herbal medicine, sometimes called botanical medicine or phytotherapy, is a type of healthcare that treats and prevents various illnesses using materials derived from plants. The practice dates back thousands of years and has its origins in the medical traditions of numerous cultures across the globe. Herbal medicine's fundamental tenets include individualization of care, prevention, and wellness as the main goals, holistic treatment, and the synergy of plant chemicals.

The holistic approach to health and healing is a cornerstone of herbal medicine. Herbal therapy attempts to treat the whole person, unlike conventional medicine, which frequently targets particular symptoms or disorders. This covers all facets of health, including mental, emotional, spiritual, and physical symptoms. Herbalists hold that plants can aid the body's natural healing process since they have an inherent capacity for self-healing. Herbal medicine aims to bring the body back into harmony and balance by considering the patient's lifestyle and general state of health.

Another fundamental idea is the synergy of plant chemicals. Herbs have many intricate chemical components that combine to provide medicinal benefits. Because of this synergy, the herb frequently has more potency than individual active components. For example, the chemicals found in garlic combine to offer antiviral, antibacterial, and anti-inflammatory properties that are stronger than those found in any one compound acting alone. This idea contradicts orthodox medicine's reductionist methodology, which favors identifying and using a single active ingredient. Herbs work synergistically to improve the body's absorption and utilization of the plant's therapeutic qualities while lowering the possibility of adverse effects.

Another fundamental tenet of herbal medicine is treatment individuation. Herbalists customize remedies based on the individual requirements of each patient, taking into account elements like age, gender, constitution, lifestyle, and the particulars of the health problem. This tailored approach recognizes that every person reacts to therapies differently and that what works for one may not work for another. By tailoring herbal treatments, herbalists can treat the underlying cause of a disease rather than just its symptoms. This idea guarantees a more focused and efficient healing strategy.

Additionally, the importance of wellness and prevention is emphasized by herbal medicine. It promotes the use of herbs to keep one's health in check and to stop illness. This proactive strategy uses herbs to boost immunity, increase vitality, and advance general health. To assist the body in handling stress and preserve homeostasis, for instance, adaptogenic herbs like ginseng and ashwagandha are utilized, which helps avoid disorders linked to stress. The emphasis on prevention is consistent with the holistic perspective on health, which places more importance on long-term wellness than temporary symptom treatment.

The fundamental tenets of herbal medicine include sustainability and reverence for the natural world. Herbalists understand the value of protecting plant diversity and applying herbs in an ecologically friendly manner. This covers the growing of therapeutic herbs, sustainable harvesting methods, and assistance with conservation initiatives. Herbal medicine fosters a polite and peaceful connection with the environment by appreciating nature and its resources.

Moreover, the foundation of herbal medicine is the idea of empowerment and education. Herbalists frequently encourage their patients to actively participate in their health by educating them about the benefits and applications of herbs. As a result of this empowerment, people are more equipped to make decisions regarding their health and well-being, which promotes a deeper comprehension of and connection to the healing process.

In summary, the fundamentals of herbal medicine emphasize a holistic approach to health, the synergistic effect of plant chemicals, customized care, preventive and wellness measures, sustainability, and patient education. These tenets provide a thorough framework for applying herbal medicine, aiming to reestablish equilibrium, assist the body's inherent healing capacity, and foster long-term health. Herbal therapy uses these ideas to offer an invaluable and efficient substitute for traditional medical practices.

Herbal preparation methods (tinctures, teas, capsules, etc.)

A vast array of procedures are employed in herbal preparation to draw out and apply the therapeutic qualities of herbs. These techniques' effectiveness, practicality, and applicability for various herbal medicines and personal preferences vary. Herbal preparations can be made into tinctures, teas, capsules, poultices, and extracts, each with specific benefits and uses.

Herbs are soaked in alcohol or a combination of alcohol and water to create tinctures, which are liquid extracts. Using this technique, the active ingredients in the herbs are efficiently extracted, becoming highly concentrated and readily absorbed by the body. Usually, tinctures are taken orally, straight under the tongue, or diluted in water or other liquids. They are a popular option for herbalists and anyone looking for reliable and robust herbal medicines because they are easy to use, have a long shelf life, and allow for accurate dosage.

Herbs can be steeped in hot water, either dry or fresh, to make teas or herbal infusions. This easy and accessible procedure requires only hot water and herbs. Herbal teas are famous for their calming and soothing properties and can be drunk hot or cold. They are accommodating for boosting general wellness, reducing intestinal discomfort, and encouraging relaxation. By combining various herbs, herbal teas can also be made to have unique flavor profiles and therapeutic benefits.

Another well-liked technique for preparing herbs is capsules, particularly for solid or bitter herbs. Herbs in powdered or encapsulated form are found in capsules, which make dosing easy and accurate. They can be taken with water or other beverages and are simple to swallow. For those who would instead take their herbs more covertly and practically—especially those who don't like the flavor of herbal tinctures or teas—capsules are the way to go. However, liquid extracts or teas may offer faster absorption or greater bioavailability than capsules.

Herbal pastes or mixtures are applied topically to the skin as poultices, which are external uses of herbs. This technique is frequently used to heal bruises, wounds, skin disorders, and muscle discomfort. Fresh or dried herbs can be crushed and combined with liquids, such as water, to make a paste for poultices. After applying the paste, the afflicted region is wrapped in a fresh cloth or bandage. Poultices can aid in the targeted relief of pain and discomfort, promote healing, and reduce inflammation.

Herbal extracts are concentrated versions of herbs usually prepared by letting the solvent from tinctures or other liquid extracts evaporate. The end product of this technique is a thick, syrupy material with a high concentration of active ingredients. Due to their potency, herbal extracts are frequently employed in tiny quantities for targeted medicinal applications or acute illnesses. They can be diluted in water for internal use, applied topically, or eaten orally. Herbal extracts offer a practical approach to delivering herbs in a concentrated form, allowing for focused and effective treatment of many health concerns.

To sum up, there are several ways to extract and use herbs' medicinal qualities through herbal preparation techniques. Every preparation method has specific benefits and uses, be it tinctures, teas, capsules, poultices, or extracts. Knowing these techniques enables people to select the best one for their requirements, preferences, and therapeutic outcomes they hope to achieve. Ultimately, a broad spectrum of people looking for natural and efficient answers to their health and wellness needs can obtain herbal therapies due to the adaptability and accessibility of herbal preparation methods.

Dosage and administration

The effectiveness and safety of herbal medicines largely depend on the remedy's dosage and administration. Herbal therapy is more flexible and customized than pharmaceutical medications, which frequently have defined dosages and administration instructions. Herbal medicines should be administered with caution, considering the potency of the plant, the patient's age, weight, overall health, and the particular health issue being treated.

The herb's strength is one significant factor when deciding on a dose. The potency and power of many herbs vary greatly; some may need more tremendous doses to produce therapeutic effects, while others may require fewer doses. Herbs with strong effects on mood and relaxation, such as valerian (Valeriana officinalis) and St. John's wort (Hypericum perforatum), may need smaller amounts to provide desirable benefits. Conversely, some herbs, such as turmeric (Curcuma longa) and ginger (Zingiber officinale), have a lower potency and may need to be taken in larger dosages to achieve the best results.

Other factors to consider are the person's age and weight. Age and weight-based adjustments may be necessary for herbal remedy dosages, as smaller people and children may need lower doses to prevent possible side effects. Similarly, older adults may require lesser dosages to have the same effects as younger people due to slower metabolisms. Speaking with a licensed herbalist or healthcare professional is crucial to determining the proper dosage for different age groups.

One's health is another essential factor to consider when choosing how much and how to administer herbal treatments. To guarantee safety and efficacy, people with specific medical problems or those on medication may need to be given extra consideration. For instance, herbs that worsen liver or kidney problems may need to be avoided by those who suffer from them, or their dosages may need to be lowered to prevent stress on the organs. Similarly, to avoid negative interactions, people using drugs that interact with herbs may need to change their dosage or stay away from particular herbs entirely.

Dosage and administration are also influenced by the particular health issue being treated. Higher doses of herbs may be necessary for acute diseases to provide relief quickly, while longer-term maintenance doses may be necessary for chronic conditions. In addition, modifications to dosage and administration may be required depending on the severity of symptoms and each patient's reaction to treatment. To get the best effects, it's critical to monitor how each person responds to herbal medicines and modify the dosage as necessary.

Depending on the intended results and the type of health problem being treated, herbal treatments can be administered orally, topically, or by inhalation. The most popular way of administration is oral, which enables systemic effects by absorbing the active ingredients into the bloodstream. Examples of oral administration include drinking herbal teas, tinctures, capsules, or extracts. Topical administration, which puts herbal remedies directly on the skin, is frequently employed to treat skin disorders, inflammation, and pain locally. Inhaling the volatile chemicals of herbs directly into the respiratory system through techniques like aromatherapy or herbal steam inhalation can be beneficial for improving mood or respiratory problems.

To sum up, dose and administration are essential factors in herbal therapy that affect the effectiveness and safety of herbal treatments. The potency, age, weight, state of health, and particular health concerns being treated are all factors that affect how much and how to administer herbal treatments. People can utilize herbal medicine to promote their health and well-being safely and effectively by carefully weighing these aspects and speaking with a licensed herbalist or healthcare provider.

Safety and Precautions

Herbal treatments include significant bioactive components that interact with the body in diverse ways; thus, safety and safeguards are crucial. Herbal medicine has many health benefits but must be used cautiously and with knowledge of hazards. Understanding safety requirements and adopting care can increase the advantages of herbal treatments while reducing side effects.

Herbal product quality and purity are safety concerns.

Buying herbs from trustworthy vendors who follow quality standards helps reduce the risk of contamination, adulteration, and mislabeling. Many choose certified organic or wildcrafted herbs because they are less likely to contain pesticides, heavy metals, etc. Standardized herbal products that have been quality-tested and verified can also guarantee potency and consistency.

Herbal treatments' safety depends on dosage and application. Take the correct dose at the right time to avoid side effects and toxicity. It's crucial to follow herbalists' or doctors' dosage recommendations and stay within them. Age, weight, health, and pre-existing medical issues or drugs should be considered while administering herbal therapies. To avoid interactions and consequences, anyone with underlying health issues or using medication should visit a doctor before commencing any herbal treatment.

Herb allergies are another safety concern. Herbal remedies are generally harmless, although some people may have allergic responses. Know your herb allergies and avoid using them if they occur. Starting with lower doses and monitoring for side effects can help discover sensitivities and prevent significant consequences.

Pharmacological qualities or drug interactions may also require precautions or contraindications for specific herbs. When taken with anticoagulants, blood-thinning herbs like ginkgo biloba or garlic may increase bleeding risk. Hormonal herbs like black cohosh and licorice root may interact with hormone-related drugs or diseases. Before utilizing herbal medicines, especially for people with health issues or who take medication, investigate herb-drug interactions and consult a doctor.

Herbal medicines may stimulate the uterine or hormonal system, which could harm pregnant or breastfeeding women. To protect mother and child, consult a doctor or herbalist before using herbal treatments during pregnancy or nursing. Professional advice is also needed because some herbs are contraindicated during pregnancy or breastfeeding.

In conclusion, herbal treatments must be used safely. Herbal medicine can be safely and effectively added to health and wellness regimens by using high-quality products, following dosage and administration guidelines, being aware of potential allergies or sensitivities, and considering individual health status and medication use. Consult with trained healthcare practitioners or herbalists and watch for side effects and interactions to ensure a happy and safe herbal remedy experience.

Potential side effects and interactions

Although herbal treatments offer many health advantages, it's crucial to understand that they may also have adverse effects and interactions, mainly if misused or in combination with other drugs or substances. It is imperative to be aware of these possible hazards for herbal medication to be used safely and effectively.

The possibility of side effects, which can vary from moderate to severe depending on the herb and individual response, is one of the main issues with herbal medicines. Common adverse effects include headaches, dizziness, allergic reactions, stomach distress, and skin irritation. Herbs like echinacea and chamomile, for instance, can trigger allergic reactions in sensitive people, and some people may experience sleepiness or gastrointestinal distress from herbs like valerian and St. John's wort. Even though side effects are usually minor and infrequent, it's essential to be aware of them and stop using the product if they do arise.

Additionally, herbal cures and medicines may interact negatively or favorably or cause inadequate responses. Drug transport systems may be interfered with, overlapping pharmacological effects may arise, or drug metabolism or absorption changes may cause these interactions. For instance, herbs like garlic, ginkgo biloba, and St. John's wort may interact with some drugs, including blood thinners, anticoagulants, and antidepressants. These interactions may result in a lower level of pharmaceutical effectiveness, a higher chance of side effects, or other unfavorable events. To prevent any drug interactions, you must speak with a healthcare professional before utilizing herbal medicines, particularly if you are already taking medication.

Some populations may be more susceptible to side effects or interactions of herbal remedies. Adverse effects may be more likely to affect children, older adults, those with existing medical issues, those who are pregnant or nursing, and people whose immune systems are impaired. For example, those who are pregnant or nursing should use caution when using herbs that are known to have uterine-stimulating or hormonal effects, as these may have an impact on the result of the pregnancy or the health of the nursing infant. In a similar vein, older adults may have slower metabolisms and be more vulnerable to adverse medication reactions.

It's crucial to utilize herbal remedies sparingly and sensibly to reduce the possibility of adverse effects and interactions. Gradually raise dosages from low starting points while watching for adverse side effects. Exercise caution when taking herbs in addition to prescription drugs or other herbal therapies. Before beginning any new treatment plan, get advice from a certified herbalist or healthcare professional. To ensure safety and avoid potential interactions, keep track of any prescriptions or supplements you take and inform your healthcare professional about any herbal remedies you intend to use.

Selecting premium herbal items from reliable vendors is also crucial to reduce the possibility of contamination, adulteration, or mislabeling. To guarantee potency and purity, look for items that have undergone quality testing and certification. Stems past their expiration date or exhibiting apparent deterioration should not be used. It is safe and useful to include herbal medicine in your regimen for health and wellness if you follow these precautions and watch out for any interactions or negative effects.

Guidelines for safe use

When adding herbal medicines to one's regimen for health and well-being, it is crucial to follow safe use guidelines to maximize benefits and reduce the possibility of negative consequences. These recommendations include a wide range of topics related to herbal medicine, such as administration, dose, sourcing, preparation, and monitoring for any possible interactions or side effects.

A basic rule of thumb is to get premium herbs from reliable vendors or cultivators. If you can, choose herbs that are wildcrafted or organic to prevent coming into contact with pesticides, herbicides, or other toxins. To guarantee that you receive the safest and most effective herbal medicines, look for products that have undergone quality, potency, and purity testing. Furthermore, be aware of any possible allergies or sensitivities to particular herbs, and refrain from using them if you have a history of allergies or unfavorable reactions.

The preparation techniques used significantly influence herbal treatments' safety and effectiveness. Whether creating teas, tinctures, capsules, extracts, or poultices, use the proper preparation methods to draw out the therapeutic qualities of the herbs. When extracting herbs with solvents or heat, exercise caution because employing too much heat or utilizing the wrong techniques might destroy the active ingredients or create toxic chemicals. To guarantee consistent and dependable outcomes, following recipes and dosage guidelines meticulously is critical.

When using herbs safely, dosage and administration are essential considerations. Begin with low dosages and raise progressively as necessary, keeping an eye out for any side effects or symptom changes. Be mindful of any interactions or contraindications with prescription drugs, over-the-counter medications, or other herbs. If you have questions, speak with a licensed healthcare professional or herbalist. Modify the dosage and administration based on individual parameters like age, weight, health state, and the particular health issue being addressed. To guarantee safety and effectiveness, herbal remedies must be customized to each person's needs.

When utilizing herbal medicines, it is imperative to monitor for potential adverse effects or interactions regularly. Watch for any modifications in symptoms or the start of new side effects, and stop using the medication if necessary. To avoid potential interactions, record all the drugs and supplements you use and let your herbalist or healthcare provider know about any herbal remedies you intend to use. Don't hesitate to seek professional advice if you have any unexpected or severe responses to herbal medicines.

Lastly, when utilizing herbal treatments, engaging in self-care and mindfulness is critical. Pay attention to your body's signals and modify your herbal regimen as necessary to enhance your general health and well-being. To maximize the benefits of herbal remedies, combine them with other holistic lifestyle practices, including a balanced diet, consistent exercise, stress reduction, and enough sleep. By following these safe usage instructions, you can take advantage of the therapeutic benefits of herbal medicine while maintaining your safety and well-being.

CHAPTER III

Top 10 Herbal Antibiotics

Garlic (Allium sativum)

Allium sativum, also known as garlic, is a multipurpose herb used medicinally for thousands of years. Garlic is well-known for its unique smell and scent but also possesses strong therapeutic qualities. The presence of flavonoids, sulfur compounds, and other bioactive substances aids this onion family member's medicinal properties. Due to its well-known antibacterial, anti-inflammatory, antioxidant, and cardiovascular properties, garlic is a widely used ingredient in food and medicine.

Garlic's antibacterial properties are among its most well-known qualities. Allicin, a sulfur-based molecule with potent antibacterial qualities, is found in garlic. Garlic is a valuable natural treatment for various ailments since allicin has been demonstrated to suppress the growth of bacteria, viruses, fungi, and parasites. Research has indicated that garlic is effective against prevalent pathogens, including but not limited to Staphylococcus aureus, Escherichia coli, Candida albicans, and certain strains that are resistant to antibiotics. Garlic's broad-spectrum antibacterial activity makes it an effective weapon against infections and a booster of the immune system.

Garlic has anti-inflammatory qualities in addition to its antibacterial ones. Numerous medical diseases, such as cancer, arthritis, and cardiovascular disease, are associated with chronic inflammation. Studies have demonstrated that chemicals found in garlic, such as diallyl sulfide and S-allyl cysteine, can lower oxidative stress and inflammation in the body. Garlic supports general health and well-being by scavenging free radicals and regulating inflammatory pathways, which help shield cells from harm.

Its antioxidant qualities further enhance garlic's health advantages. Unstable chemicals called free radicals can harm cells and accelerate aging and disease processes. Antioxidants found in garlic, including flavonoids, selenium, and vitamin C, work to scavenge free radicals and stop oxidative damage. Garlic enhances the immune system, brain, and cardiovascular health by lowering oxidative stress and inflammation. Frequent garlic consumption may help reduce the risk of developing chronic illnesses like Alzheimer's disease, heart disease, and several types of cancer.

The cardiovascular health advantages of garlic are also widely recognized. Studies have shown that garlic may help lower blood pressure, cut cholesterol, and enhance circulation. Garlic's capacity to lower blood pressure, stop platelet aggregation, and control lipid metabolism is thought to be responsible for these benefits. By improving cardiovascular health, garlic may help reduce the risk of heart attack, stroke, and other cardiovascular events. One way to keep your heart healthy and prevent cardiovascular disease is to include garlic in a balanced diet and lifestyle.

Garlic comes in a variety of forms and dishes that can be eaten. Dicing, mashing, or chopping fresh garlic cloves adds taste and health benefits to food. The most effective form of garlic is raw because heat can deactivate some health-promoting ingredients. For individuals who want a more handy and concentrated dose, garlic supplements are now available in the form of capsules, tablets, and extracts. Standardized dosages of garlic extract are frequently included in these supplements, which facilitates the achievement of therapeutic effects. Furthermore, aged garlic extract has improved bioavailability and may provide additional health advantages because it is fermented.

To sum up, garlic is a fantastic herb with various therapeutic benefits. It is a beneficial addition to culinary and pharmaceutical regimens due to its antibacterial, anti-inflammatory, antioxidant, and cardiovascular properties. Garlic has been used for generations to promote well-being and vigor. It offers several health benefits, either ingested fresh, as a supplement, or in extract form. People can use the medicinal properties of this age-old herb to enhance their general health and well-being by including garlic in a balanced diet and way of life.

Echinacea (Echinacea spp.)

Echinacea is a genus of herbaceous flowering plants native to North America. Native American cultures have long utilized echinacea species, also referred to as coneflowers, for their therapeutic benefits. Today, echinacea is a well-liked herbal medicine for various health ailments due to its generally acknowledged immune-boosting and anti-inflammatory properties.

Echinacea's immunomodulatory action is one of its main characteristics. Bioactive substances in echinacea, such as flavonoids, polysaccharides, and alkamides, boost the immune system and improve the body's natural defenses against illnesses. Studies have shown that echinacea can improve phagocytosis, raise white blood cell synthesis, and stimulate immune cells, including natural killer cells and macrophages. Echinacea is frequently used to prevent and treat respiratory infections, colds, the flu, and other common ailments by boosting immune function.

Echinacea has immune-boosting and anti-inflammatory qualities. Numerous medical disorders, such as autoimmune illnesses, allergies, and chronic pain, are linked to chronic inflammation. Alkamides and caffeic acid derivatives, two substances found in echinacea, block inflammatory pathways and lower the release of pro-inflammatory cytokines. Echinacea reduces inflammation, which helps to improve general health and well-being and lessen symptoms related to inflammatory disorders.

Common uses for echinacea include treating and preventing upper respiratory tract infections, including the flu and the common cold. According to research, echinacea may lessen the intensity and length of respiratory infection symptoms such as sore throat, cough, congestion, and exhaustion. Improving immune response and reducing vulnerability to infections might also aid in preventing recurrent infections. Echinacea is frequently taken to maintain immune function during cold and flu season, either at the onset of symptoms or as a preventive approach.

Echinacea comes in a variety of forms and preparations for eating. Supplements containing echinacea, such as extracts, tinctures, capsules, and pills, are easily accessible and user-friendly. Standardized dosages of echinacea extract are frequently included in these supplements, which facilitates the achievement of therapeutic effects. Another well-liked preparation technique is echinacea tea, created from dried echinacea roots, leaves, or flowers. For added advantages, echinacea tea is sometimes prepared with other immune-boosting herbs, including elderberry, ginger, and licorice. It can be taken hot or cold.

When buying echinacea products, use premium supplements from reliable suppliers to guarantee effectiveness and purity. Seek items that have undergone quality testing and have been standardized to include particular active component concentrations. Furthermore, be aware of any possible echinacea allergies or sensitivities, particularly in people who have previously experienced allergies to plants in the Asteraceae family.

To summarize, echinacea is a multipurpose herb with anti-inflammatory, solid, and immune-boosting qualities. It is an effective treatment and prevention method for common illnesses, including the flu, colds, and respiratory infections, because of its capacity to boost immune system activity and lower inflammation. Echinacea has been used for generations to boost immune function and general well-being. It can be taken as a supplement, tea, or extract, offering various health advantages. People can use the therapeutic properties of echinacea to stay well and resistant to illnesses and diseases by including it in a balanced diet and way of life.

Goldenseal (Hydrastis canadensis)

North American goldenseal (Hydrastis canadensis) is regarded for its therapeutic benefits and traditional applications by indigenous peoples. This herb, also known as yellow root or orange root, has been used medicinally by Native Americans like the Cherokee and Iroquois. Goldenseal includes bioactive alkaloids such as berberine, hydrastine, and canadine, which are medicinal. Its antimicrobial, anti-inflammatory, and immune-modulating characteristics make goldenseal a popular herbal therapy for many health ailments.

Antimicrobial activity is a prominent goldenseal property. Berberine, one of goldenseal's primary alkaloids, has been widely examined for its broad- spectrum antibacterial activities. Goldenseal is a powerful natural infection medicine because berberine inhibits bacteria, viruses, fungi, and parasites. Studies have shown goldenseal's effectiveness against Staphylococcus aureus, E. coli, Candida albicans, and Helicobacter pylori. Due to its antibacterial characteristics, goldenseal fights infections, boosts immunity, and promotes wellness.

Goldenseal is antibacterial and anti-inflammatory.

Chronic inflammation can cause arthritis, allergies, and intestinal issues. Berberine and hydrastine in goldenseal decrease inflammation and alter immunological function. Goldenseal reduces pro-inflammatory cytokines and inflammatory pathways to relieve symptoms and improve healing.

Goldenseal is used to boost immunity and prevent infections. Its immuno-modulating properties boost the body's pathogen defenses and immune function. Goldenseal is used during cold and flu season or at the first sign of symptoms to enhance immunity and shorten illnesses. It treats respiratory, nasal, urinary, and gastrointestinal diseases due to its antibacterial and anti-inflammatory properties.

Different goldenseal formulations are available for

eating. Goldenseal capsules, pills, tinctures, and extracts are readily accessible and easy to use. Goldenseal extract is usually standardized in these supplements, making therapeutic benefits easier to accomplish. Another popular preparation is dried goldenseal root or leaf tea. Goldenseal tea is prepared with echinacea, ginger, and elderberry for increased immunity and served hot or cold.

To ensure efficacy and purity, pick high-quality goldenseal pills from trusted providers. Choose quality-tested items with particular active component concentrations. Goldenseal may interact with drugs and other herbs, so consult a doctor before using it, especially if you have a health problem or are taking medication.

Lastly, goldenseal is a powerful antibacterial, anti-inflammatory, and immune-modulating plant. Its capacity to fight infections, reduce inflammation, and boost immunity makes it a flexible and valuable herbal therapy for many health disorders. Goldenseal has been used for generations as a supplement, tea, or extract to boost health and vigor. Adding goldenseal to a balanced diet and lifestyle can improve health.

Ginger (Zingiber officinale)

Southeast Asian native ginger (Zingiber officinale) is a blooming plant that has long been valued for its culinary and therapeutic uses. Traditional medical systems like Ayurveda and Traditional Chinese Medicine (TCM) have traditionally used this herbaceous perennial. Ginger's flavor and therapeutic properties are attributed to its bioactive components, including zingerone, shogaol, and gingerol. Ginger is a popular and adaptable herbal medicine because of its well-known anti-inflammatory, antioxidant, digestive, and immune-boosting qualities.

Ginger's anti-inflammatory effects are among its main advantages. Numerous medical diseases, including arthritis, digestive issues, and cardiovascular disease, have been linked to chronic inflammation. Studies have demonstrated that chemicals found in ginger, such as gingerol and shogaol, block inflammatory pathways and decrease the generation of pro-inflammatory cytokines. Ginger reduces inflammation, which helps to improve general health and well-being and lessen symptoms related to inflammatory disorders.

Ginger is frequently used to promote gastrointestinal health and ease digestion-related discomfort. Its antispasmodic and carminative qualities aid digestion, relieve bloating and gas, and relax intestinal muscles. To help with the breakdown and absorption of nutrients, ginger increases the production of gastric juices and digestive enzymes. Ginger is frequently used during pregnancy to treat motion sickness, morning sickness, nausea, and indigestion. It is a well-liked treatment for discomfort and digestive problems because of its calming effects on the stomach.

Ginger has digestive and anti-inflammatory benefits, but it also has antioxidant qualities. Unstable chemicals called free radicals can harm cells and accelerate the aging and disease processes. Antioxidants found in ginger, such as zingerone and gingerol, aid in scavenging free radicals and halting oxidative damage. Ginger helps the immune, brain, and cardiovascular systems by lowering oxidative stress. Frequent ginger consumption may help reduce the risk of developing chronic illnesses like Alzheimer's disease, heart disease, and some types of cancer.

Additionally prized for its immune-boosting qualities is ginger. According to studies, ginger can improve the body's natural defenses against infections and boost immunological function. Ginger is a valuable natural treatment for preventing and treating infections because it includes bioactive components with antibacterial and antiviral properties, such as zingerone and gingerol. During the cold and flu season, ginger is typically taken as a prophylactic or as soon as symptoms appear to boost immune function and lessen the intensity and length of illnesses.

Ginger can be consumed in a variety of forms and recipes. For flavor and health advantages, fresh ginger root can be diced, sliced, or grated and added to food. The most effective form of ginger is raw because heat might inactivate some of its health-promoting ingredients. For people who would instead take their supplements in a more handy and concentrated form, there are now capsules, pills, and extracts of ginger available. Standardized dosages of ginger extract are frequently included in these supplements, which facilitates the achievement of therapeutic effects. Another well-liked preparation technique is ginger tea, brewed from either fresh or dried ginger root. Ginger tea is a hot or cold beverage that tastes great with other immune-stimulating herbs like mint, lemon, and honey.

Ginger is a multipurpose herb with digestive solid, anti-inflammatory, antioxidant, and immune-boosting qualities. Its beneficial effects on immunological function, inflammation reduction, and digestive discomfort make it a tremendous herbal therapy for various ailments. Ginger has been used for generations to support energy and well-being. It can be ingested fresh, as a supplement, or in tea. People can utilize ginger's therapeutic properties to enhance their general health and well-being by including it in a balanced diet and way of life.

Turmeric (Curcuma longa)

South Asian rhizomatous herbaceous perennial turmeric (Curcuma longa) is known for its bright golden-yellow hue and several health advantages. This spice has been utilized in Ayurvedic and Chinese medicine for millennia for its therapeutic effects. The bioactive component curcumin gives turmeric various medicinal properties. Turmeric is a helpful herbal medicine since curcumin is an antioxidant and anti-inflammatory.

Turmeric has potent anti-inflammatory effects. Arthritis, cardiovascular disease, and neurological illnesses are linked to chronic inflammation. Curcumin in turmeric inhibits inflammatory pathways and decreases pro-inflammatory cytokines, reducing inflammation and promoting healing. Turmeric supplements lower inflammation markers and relieve symptoms of inflammatory disorders like arthritis and irritable bowel syndrome, according to research.

Turmeric is revered for its antioxidants. Unstable free radicals harm cells and cause aging and disease. Curcumin neutralizes oxidative stress and free radicals. Turmeric reduces oxidative damage and inflammation, improving heart, brain, and immunological health. Regular turmeric use may reduce the risk of heart disease, Alzheimer's, and certain malignancies.

Turmeric is used to relieve stomach discomfort and support gastrointestinal health. Its carminative and anti-inflammatory effects soothe the digestive tract, reduce gas and bloating, and aid digestion. Turmeric increases bile production, which breaks down and absorbs fats and minerals. Indigestion, bloating, gas, and heartburn are treated with turmeric. Supporting digestive health makes it a popular therapy for gastrointestinal disorders and discomfort.

Turmeric has anti-inflammatory, antioxidant, digestive, antibacterial, and immune-boosting effects. Curcumin inhibits bacteria, viruses, fungi, and parasites, making it an effective natural infection treatment. Turmeric boosts the body's natural defenses against infections, preventing disease and supporting immunological health. Turmeric is used throughout cold and flu season or at the first sign of symptoms to enhance immunity and shorten illnesses.

Many turmeric formulations are available for eating. Grated, sliced, or diced fresh turmeric root adds taste and therapeutic advantages to meals. Heat deactivates part of turmeric's benefits. Thus, raw turmeric is the strongest. Turmeric capsules, pills, and extracts are available for convenience and concentration. Standardized curcumin dosages in these supplements make therapeutic effects simpler. Popular preparations include turmeric tea made from fresh or dried turmeric root. Hot or cold turmeric tea is commonly made with immune-boosting herbs, including ginger, cinnamon, and lemon.

Finally, turmeric has potent anti-inflammatory, antioxidant, digestive, antibacterial, and immune-boosting qualities. Its ability to reduce inflammation, enhance digestive health, and boost immunological function makes it a beneficial herbal therapy for many ailments. Turmeric has been used for generations to boost health and energy when ingested fresh, as a supplement, or in tea. When added to a balanced diet and lifestyle, turmeric can boost health and well-being.

Oregano (Origanum vulgare) Properties, uses, and preparations

The Mediterranean herb oregano (Origanum vulgare) is fragrant and tasty, and it is used in cooking and medicine. This mint family perennial herb has been utilized in Ayurveda and Mediterranean folk medicine for millennia for its medicinal properties. Bioactive chemicals like carvacrol, thymol, and rosmarinic acid give oregano its characteristic fragrance and powerful therapeutic properties. Oregano is a popular herbal treatment due to its antibacterial, anti-inflammatory, antioxidant, and digestive qualities.

A fundamental property of oregano is its antibacterial capabilities. Oregano's principal bioactive components, carvacrol and thymol, inhibit bacteria, fungi, and parasites. The plant leaves yield antibacterial properties, making oregano oil a popular natural cure for numerous diseases. Studies have shown oregano's effectiveness against Staphylococcus aureus, E. coli, Candida albicans, and Aspergillus spp. Its broad-spectrum antibacterial action makes oregano helpful in fighting infections and improving health.

Oregano is antibacterial, anti-inflammatory, and antioxidant. Inflammation and oxidative stress are associated with arthritis, cardiovascular disease, and neurological illnesses. Rosmarinic acid and flavonoids in oregano decrease inflammation and neutralize free radicals. Oregano boosts heart, brain, and immunological health by suppressing inflammatory pathways and scavenging free radicals. Regular oregano ingestion may reduce chronic illness risk and enhance longevity.

Oregano is used to relieve digestive discomfort and support gastrointestinal health. Its carminative and digestive characteristics soothe the digestive tract, reduce gas and bloating, and aid digestion. Oregano boosts digestive enzymes and stomach secretions, which help absorb nutrition. Dried oregano leaves make tea for indigestion, bloating, gas, and heartburn. Due to its digestive health benefits, oregano is often used to treat GI disorders.

Oregano comes in several forms. Fresh or dried oregano leaves bring flavor and medicine to recipes. Concentrated oregano oil from the plant's leaves is utilized for its antibacterial and medicinal properties. Oregano capsules, pills, and extracts are offered for convenience and concentration. Standardized oregano extract concentrations in these supplements make therapeutic effects simpler. Oregano tea made from dried leaves is also popular. Oregano tea is made with thyme, sage, and lemon for enhanced immunity and served hot or cold.

Oregano is a multipurpose plant with potent antibacterial, anti-inflammatory, antioxidant, and digestive activities. It is a helpful herbal medicine for many health concerns since it fights infections, reduces inflammation, and supports digestion. Oregano has been used for ages to improve health and vigor as a culinary herb, essential oil, supplement, or tea. People can benefit from its healing properties by adding oregano to a healthy diet and lifestyle.

CHAPTER IV

Herbal Antibiotics for Common Ailments

Colds, flu, bronchitis

Antibiotics made from herbs have long been used as efficient treatments for common illnesses, including the flu, bronchitis, and colds. These all-natural substitutes support the body's immune system and manage symptoms comprehensively. Several herbs are effective partners in the fight against respiratory infections because of their antibacterial, anti-inflammatory, and immune-boosting qualities.

One of the most well-known herbal antibiotics is echinacea, which is highly valued for its ability to strengthen immunity. This herb helps the body's defense mechanisms against bacteria and viruses and promotes the generation of white blood cells. Common uses for echinacea include upper respiratory tract infections, the flu, and cold prevention. It is a well-liked option during the cold and flu season because of its capacity to lessen the intensity and length of symptoms.

Ginger is another solid natural antibiotic that has immune-modulating and anti-inflammatory qualities. Cough, congestion, and sore throat are some symptoms of respiratory infections that ginger helps relieve. Its warming qualities ease bronchial spasms and congestion in the chest while also enhancing circulation. Made from fresh or dried ginger root, ginger tea can be frequently drunk to enhance immunological function and is a relaxing cure for respiratory pain.

Furthermore, oregano is highly valued for its antibacterial properties, especially in its essential oil, which has vital ingredients including thymol and carvacrol; among the many pathogens that oregano oil effectively combats are bacteria, viruses, and fungi. It can be applied locally or taken internally to treat respiratory infections and ease symptoms like inflammation of the bronchi and sinuses, coughing, and fever. Inhaling steam or using a diffuser with oregano oil might assist in relieving congestion and supporting respiratory comfort.

Garlic is also a potent natural antibiotic with broad-spectrum antibacterial qualities. Garlic contains a sulfur molecule called allicin, which has strong antiviral, antibacterial, and antifungal properties. Eating raw garlic or taking supplements containing garlic helps strengthen the immune system and prevent illnesses. It's usual practice to use garlic to treat and prevent respiratory infections, such as sinusitis, pneumonia, and bronchitis.

Another herbal treatment frequently used for respiratory conditions is eucalyptus, which has antibacterial, expectorant, and decongestant qualities. Cineole, a substance found in eucalyptus essential oil, aids in clearing congestion and releasing mucus. Eucalyptus oil vapors are a well-liked treatment for colds, flu, and bronchitis because they facilitate breathing and calm irritated respiratory tracts.

It's essential to speak with a skilled herbalist or healthcare provider before utilizing herbal antibiotics for common respiratory infections, particularly if you have underlying medical disorders or are on medication. Herbal treatments can interfere with some drugs and may not be appropriate for everyone, even though they provide a natural substitute for conventional antibiotics. Utilizing premium herbs from reliable suppliers is critical to guarantee potency and purity.

In summary, herbal antibiotics offer efficient and all-natural treatments for common respiratory conditions like the flu, bronchitis, and colds. Herbs with antibacterial, anti-inflammatory, and immune-boosting qualities include echinacea, ginger, oregano, garlic, and eucalyptus. These properties can aid in the relief of symptoms and promote healing. Including these herbal remedies in your wellness regimen may improve your body's natural defenses against infections and support respiratory health.

Cuts, burns, acne

Herbal antibiotics are a safe, all-natural way to treat common illnesses, and using particular herbs in recipes can help treat a variety of disorders more precisely. Many herbs are excellent friends in the fight against infections and in enhancing general well-being because of their strong antibacterial, anti-inflammatory, and immune-boosting qualities.

Garlic is one such herb well-known for its broad-spectrum antibacterial properties. Allicin, a sulfur-based molecule found in garlic, has strong antiviral, antibacterial, and antifungal effects. Eating raw garlic or taking supplements containing garlic helps strengthen the immune system and prevent illnesses. Garlic-infused honey is a popular dish that uses raw garlic cloves steeped in honey to make a solid, immune-boosting tonic. Colds, sore throats, and respiratory infections respond best to this treatment.

Another plant frequently utilized for its immune-boosting properties is echinacea. Echinacea stimulates white blood cell production and helps the body's defense mechanisms against bacteria and viruses. Dried echinacea roots or leaves are used to make echinacea tea, a well-liked treatment for upper respiratory tract infections, colds, and flu. Other immune-stimulating herbs like ginger, lemon, and honey can be added to the tea to increase its effectiveness and offer further symptom alleviation.

Oregano is highly valued for its antibacterial properties, especially in its essential oil with vital ingredients, including thymol and carvacrol. To treat infections and alleviate symptoms like cough, sinus congestion, and bronchi inflammation, oregano oil can be used topically or consumed. A primary method for making oregano oil involves soaking dried oregano leaves in olive oil for a few weeks and then straining the concoction to remove the oil. Cuts, wounds, and skin infections can benefit from applying this homemade oregano oil as a natural antibiotic ointment.

Because of its well-known anti-inflammatory and immune-stimulating qualities, ginger is a valuable plant for stomach problems and respiratory infections. A relaxing cure for cough, congestion, and sore throat is ginger tea, which is prepared from fresh or dried ginger root. Ginger tea can be made even more immune-boosting and symptom-relieving by adding other herbs like turmeric, cinnamon, and lemon. Another use for ginger is in preparing ginger syrup, made by simmering fresh ginger root in water and sugar to produce a thick syrup that may be used as an immune-boosting addition to teas, smoothies, or desserts.

Eucalyptus is frequently used to treat respiratory conditions because of its expectorant, antimicrobial, and decongestant qualities. Eucalyptus essential oil can be mixed with steam inhalations or diffusers to relieve respiratory distress and calm irritated respiratory tracts. To inhale eucalyptus steam, mix a few drops of eucalyptus oil with a bowl of hot water, cover your head with a towel, and take deep breaths of the steam for a few minutes. This treatment helps facilitate respiratory comfort, reduce sinus pressure, and eliminate congestion.

To sum up, several herbs and recipes provide targeted relief for common ailments ranging from digestive problems to respiratory infections. Herbal therapies such as garlic-infused honey, echinacea tea, oregano oil, ginger syrup, and eucalyptus steam inhalation can support general well-being by enhancing the immune system and easing symptoms. You can use the natural therapeutic properties of these herbs and recipes to improve your overall wellness regimen and promote your health and well-being.

Food poisoning, stomach flu

Herbal antibiotics are natural and effective treatments for common illnesses, including food poisoning and stomach flu. They offer relief from symptoms and promote recovery without the need for synthetic medicines, making them an alternative to conventional methods of treatment. These natural alternatives use medicinal plants' power to treat infections, alleviate digestive distress, and promote the health of the gastrointestinal tract.

Ginger, scientifically known as Zingiber officinale, is widely recognized as a beneficial herb for treating gastrointestinal disorders. As a result of its digestive and anti-nausea effects, ginger has been utilized for ages in traditional medical practices such as Ayurveda and Traditional Chinese Medicine (TCM). Ginger is a source of bioactive chemicals such as gingerol and school, which have been shown to reduce nausea and vomiting, stimulate digestion, and calm the muscles of the gastrointestinal tract. In addition to relieving symptoms of food poisoning and stomach flu, such as nausea, vomiting, diarrhea, and abdominal discomfort, drinking ginger tea or chewing on fresh ginger slices can also relieve these symptoms.

Peppermint, also known as Mentha piperita, is another herb frequently used to treat gastrointestinal disorders. Menthol, found in peppermint, is a chemical shown to exhibit antispasmodic and analgesic effects on the digestive tract. It is possible to alleviate the symptoms of food poisoning and stomach flu by drinking peppermint tea or taking peppermint capsules. These symptoms include cramping, bloating, and indigestion. A topical application of peppermint oil that has been diluted and applied to the abdomen can also assist in alleviating discomfort in the gastrointestinal tract and reduce gas and bloating.

Regarding the digestive tract, chamomile, also known as Matricaria chamomilla, is well regarded for its relaxing and anti-inflammatory properties. Flavonoids with anti-inflammatory properties, such as apigenin and chamazulene, are found in chamomile tea. These flavonoids assist in reducing inflammation, soothe inflamed mucous membranes and aid digestion. Chamomile tea can help alleviate symptoms of food poisoning and stomach flu, such as nausea, cramping, and diarrhea. Chamomile tea can also boost the immune system. Additionally, chamomile tea can assist in relaxing the body and ensure a peaceful night's sleep, both of which are necessary for the recovery process following gastrointestinal ailments.

In addition to being a beneficial herb for fighting off infections, such as those that cause food poisoning and stomach flu, echinacea (Echinacea spp.) is well-known for its immune-enhancing characteristics. The consumption of echinacea raises the number of white blood cells in the body, strengthening the body's natural defenses against infectious agents. The use of echinacea tea or supplements can assist in the enhancement of the immune system, as well as the reduction of the severity and length of symptoms that are generally associated with gastrointestinal illnesses. Echinacea can improve immune function and reduce susceptibility to pathogens, which are essential in preventing recurring infections.

In addition to being a powerful antimicrobial herb, garlic, also known as Allium sativum, can be used to treat the microorganisms responsible for food poisoning and stomach flu. On the other hand, garlic includes allicin, a sulfur component with antibacterial, antiviral, and antifungal properties that are broad-spectrum. Consumption of raw garlic or garlic supplements can enhance the immune system and assist in the battle against illnesses. The symptoms of gastrointestinal infections, such as nausea, vomiting, diarrhea, and abdominal discomfort, can also be alleviated with the help of garlic. Adding raw garlic to dishes such as stews, soups, and other cuisines can provide additional advantages to the immune system and provide antibacterial protection.

These individual herbs can be beneficial in treating food poisoning and stomach flu, and herbal mixtures and formulations can also be effective in treating these conditions. A combination of ginger, peppermint, chamomile, and echinacea, for instance, can provide complete relief from symptoms while supporting immune function and digestive health. The use of herbal formulations specifically developed for gastrointestinal difficulties, such as tinctures or capsules containing a combination of digestive herbs, can also be effective in reducing symptoms and encouraging healing.

Contacting a skilled healthcare physician or herbalist before utilizing herbal antibiotics for food poisoning and stomach flu is vital. This is especially important if you have any preexisting health concerns or are taking any medications. Even though herbal treatments provide natural alternatives to conventional drugs, they may not be appropriate for everyone and may interact with specific medications. In addition, it is essential to use herbs of superior quality that come from reliable sources to guarantee their potency and purity.

In conclusion, herbal antibiotics offer natural and efficient treatments for relatively frequent gastrointestinal conditions, such as food poisoning and stomach flu. Herbs such as ginger, peppermint, chamomile, echinacea, and garlic are just a few examples of herbs with potent antibacterial, anti- inflammatory, and immune-enhancing characteristics. These herbs can help reduce symptoms and aid healing. Incorporating these herbs into your wellness regimen allows you to harness the healing power of nature, which in turn supports your digestive health and overall well-being naturally.

Urinary Tract Infections

Urinary tract infections (UTIs) are widespread bacterial illnesses that primarily afflict women and impact millions of individuals globally each year. Although UTIs are frequently treated with antibiotics, abuse of these drugs has resulted in antibiotic resistance and unfavorable side effects. Without synthetic medications, herbal antibiotics provide safe, natural alternatives for treating urinary tract infections (UTIs), relieving symptoms, and enhancing urinary tract health.

Cranberry (Vaccinium macrocarpon) is one of the most popular herbs used to treat UTIs. Proanthocyanidins in cranberries inhibit bacteria like Escherichia coli (E. coli) from sticking to the urinary tract walls and causing infection. Cranberry juice or supplements might lessen the chance of a urinary tract infection (UTI) and ease symptoms, including burning, discomfort, and urgency when urinating. Because cranberry supplements come in various forms, such as concentrated extracts, pills, and capsules, it is simple and handy to incorporate them into a daily routine.

Another herb frequently used for UTIs is dandelion (Taraxacum officinale), which has both diuretic and antibacterial qualities. Supplements or tea made from dandelion leaves can stimulate urine production and remove bacteria from the urinary tract. Dandelion root also has substances that aid in liver detoxification and function, which can improve the body's capacity to get rid of pollutants and fend against infections. Regularly consuming dandelion tea can lower the incidence of recurring UTIs and assist in preserving urinary tract health.

Thanks to its well-known antibacterial and diuretic properties, uva ursi (Arctostaphylos uva-ursi) is a valuable herb for treating urinary tract infections. Arbutin, a substance found in uva ursi, is transformed by the body into hydroquinone and then eliminated in the urine, where it functions as an antibacterial agent. Inhibiting the growth of bacteria in the urinary tract and reducing symptoms of a urinary tract infection (UTI), including discomfort, burning, and frequent urination, can be achieved by consuming uva ursi tea or supplements. However, if taken in large amounts or for an extended length of time, uva ursi can have adverse effects like nausea, vomiting, and liver damage. As such, it should only be used under the supervision of a healthcare professional.

Solidago virgaurea, or goldenrod, is a highly valued herb for urinary tract infections due to its diuretic and anti-inflammatory characteristics. Flavonoids and saponins found in goldenrod enhance urinary tract health by reducing inflammation. Goldenrod tea and supplements can help relieve burning, discomfort, and urgency when urinating—all signs of urinary tract infections. Goldenrod can also aid in removing pathogens from the urinary tract and encourage the healing of irritated tissues. To completely treat the symptoms of a urinary tract infection, goldenrod is frequently used with other herbs like cranberry and dandelion.

Herbal formulations and combinations, in addition to these single herbs, can be helpful in the treatment of urinary tract infections. For instance, cranberries, dandelion, uva ursi, and goldenrod can offer complete symptom alleviation while treating the infection's underlying cause. Additionally helpful in reducing symptoms and enhancing urinary tract health are herbal formulations created especially for UTIs, such as tinctures or capsules that contain a combination of herbs that support the urinary system.

It's essential to speak with a licensed healthcare professional or herbalist before utilizing herbal antibiotics for UTIs, particularly if you have underlying medical concerns or are taking medication. Herbal medicines can interfere with some prescriptions and may not be suited for everyone, even though they provide natural alternatives to conventional drugs. To guarantee potency and purity, utilizing premium herbs from reliable suppliers is critical.

Finally, herbal antibiotics offer safe, healthy substitutes for prescription drugs when treating urinary tract infections. Herbs having strong antibacterial, anti-inflammatory, and diuretic qualities that can aid with symptoms and support urinary tract health include cranberries, dandelion, uva ursi, and goldenrod. You may use these herbs' natural healing properties to enhance your urinary system's health and well-being. Just incorporate them into your daily wellness practice.

CHAPTER V

Creating Your Herbal Medicine Cabinet

Essential Herbs to Keep on Hand Detailed list and descriptions

Keeping necessary herbs on hand is a good idea to preserve your general health and well-being. These herbs can be helpful allies in supporting several elements of health and have a wide range of applications, from culinary to medicinal. This is a comprehensive list of necessary herbs to always have on hand, complete with usage and health benefits notes.

Basil (Ocimum basilicum) is a fragrant plant frequently used in Asian and Mediterranean cooking. Its sweet, somewhat spicy flavor is a result of its abundance of anti-inflammatory and antioxidant-rich ingredients. Basil helps lower inflammation and support digestive health. It can also be infused into oil for aromatherapy or applied topically as a natural insect repellant.

Rosemary (Rosmarinus officinalis): A woody herb with a strong flavor and perfume akin to pine, rosemary is frequently used in cooking to enhance the flavor of meats, vegetables, and bread. It is advantageous for boosting immune system performance and avoiding infections because of its high antioxidant content and antibacterial qualities. For topical application, rosemary can also be blended into oil to reduce muscle soreness and enhance circulation.

Thyme (Thymus vulgaris): A flavorful and adaptable herb often used in soups, stews, and meat preparations, thyme is also a natural topical antibacterial for cuts and skin infections. Thymol, an antibacterial and expectorant chemical, is present in thyme, making it helpful in treating coughs and respiratory infections.

Petroselinum crispum, or parsley, is a bright, delicious herb that tastes mildly of pepper. It can be used as a flavoring or garnish in various recipes. Because of its abundance of vitamins, minerals, and antioxidants, it is suitable for detoxification and general health support. In addition, parsley can be added to tea or applied topically to relieve skin irritation and improve breath.

Mint (Mentha spp.): A cooling herb with a minty flavor, mint is often used in teas, salads, and desserts. Because of its analgesic and antispasmodic qualities, menthol can help relieve headaches, nausea, and intestinal discomfort. Mint can also be utilized in aromatherapy or infused into oil to help with relaxation and focus.

Lavender (Lavandula spp.): Lavender is a fragrant and pleasant flowery scent often used in herbal medicine, aromatherapy, and cuisine. Its relaxing and sedative qualities make it advantageous for lowering tension, anxiety, and sleeplessness. In addition, lavender can be applied directly or blended into oil to treat pain, inflammation, and skin irritation.

Allium sativum, or garlic, is an aromatic herb with a robust and unique flavor frequently used in cooking to give food more flavor and depth. It can help prevent infections and enhance immune function by including allicin, which has antibacterial solid and immune-boosting characteristics. Additionally, garlic can be applied topically to treat wounds and skin infections as a natural antiseptic.

Ginger (Zingiber officinale): Frequently utilized in teas, herbal medicines, and cuisine, ginger is a warm, citrusy, and spicy herb. Because it includes gingerol's anti-inflammatory and digestive components, it can help with indigestion, nausea, and menstrual cramps. In addition, ginger can be applied topically or incorporated into oil to reduce muscle soreness and enhance circulation.

Curcuma longa, or turmeric, is a bright yellow plant that tastes warm and slightly bitter. It is frequently added to smoothies, soups, and curries. Turmeric helps reduce inflammation, promote joint health, and prevent chronic diseases because it includes curcumin, a substance with potent anti-inflammatory and antioxidant properties. Turmeric can also be used topically or blended into oil to reduce pain and improve skin health.

Matricaria chamomilla, also known as chamomile, is a mild, calming herb with a sweet, flowery flavor frequently added to teas, tinctures, and cosmetics products. Because of its anti-inflammatory and soothing qualities, it can help ease intestinal discomfort, anxiety, and stress. In addition, chamomile can be applied topically or blended into oil to treat sunburn, inflammation, and skin irritation.

In summary, having the necessary herbs is an easy yet powerful method to support well-being. Herbs that are adaptable and can be used in cooking, drinks, aromatherapy, and herbal medicines include basil, rosemary, thyme, parsley, mint, lavender, garlic, ginger, turmeric, and chamomile. By integrating these herbs into your daily regimen, you may utilize their distinct tastes, scents, and therapeutic qualities to enhance your general well-being and energy levels.

Tools and Supplies Needed Equipment for preparation and storage

Having the appropriate tools and supplies is necessary when effectively preparing and preserving herbs and herbal treatments. Possessing the proper equipment means that you will be able to organize and preserve herbs in a safe and effective manner, regardless of whether you are harvesting them from your garden or purchasing them from a store. The following is an in-depth summary of the equipment and supplies required to prepare and preserve herbal remedies.

When it comes to harvesting herbs, whether cultivating them in your garden or picking them from the wild, you will want a few essential pieces of equipment to gather them efficiently. Some examples are garden shears or scissors for cutting herbs, a trowel or other digging instrument for harvesting roots and a basket or container for collecting the herbs that have been picked. It is essential to make use of tools that are both clean and sharp to avoid causing any harm to the plants and to guarantee a clean harvest.

Drying herbs is a usual practice to preserve them for later use. Drying equipment is used for this purpose. To successfully dry herbs, you will want sufficient airflow and a low humidity level. It would help if you used an herb drying rack or screen since it allows air to circulate the herbs while preventing them from coming into contact with one another. Alternatively, you can hang bundles of herbs in an area that has adequate ventilation by hanging them upside down. In addition to a drying rack or hanging space, you might also want a dehydrator to dry herbs quickly and effectively. This is especially true if you reside in an area that experiences high levels of humidity.

Containers for storage: once herbs have been dried, they must be stored appropriately to keep their flavor and potency intact. Jars made of glass with airtight lids are the best containers for storing dry herbs since they shield the herbs from air, light, and moisture. Mason jars and other glass containers with lids that can be screwed on are excellent choices for this use. To maintain a record of the freshness of the herbs, it is essential to label the jars with the name of the herb and the date that they were harvested. When storing powdered herbs or herbal blends, portable containers with lids that may be sealed securely are accessible and practical.

It would help to have the right equipment to grind dried herbs into powder or blend them. If you plan to do either, you must have the equipment. The traditional method of crushing herbs into powder is accomplished using a mortar and pestle, which allows you to regulate the texture and consistency of the finished product. An electric spice or coffee grinder is another option that can be utilized to grind more significant quantities of spices or achieve a more precise grinding. In addition, mixing bowls and spoons is necessary for blending herbs to develop individualized formulations or herbal treatments.

Tinctures are concentrated herbal extracts from steeping herbs in either alcohol or glycerin. Tinctures are available for purchase. It is necessary to have glass bottles or jars with lids that can be sealed securely to store the finished product while making tinctures. Regarding tinctures, amber glass bottles are the most favored option because they shield the contents from the effects of light loss. In addition, you will require a graduated cylinder or a measuring scale to measure the ratios of the herb to the liquid correctly. Additionally, you will need a cheesecloth or a filter with a fine mesh to remove the plant material after it has allowed the herbs to steep.

Equipment Used for Infusions and Decoctions Infusions and decoctions are herbal preparations created by steeping herbs in hot water at a low temperature. If you want to make infusions, you will need glass teapots or jars that are heat-resistant and have lids so that you can cover the infusion while it is steeping. When making decoctions, which require herbs to be simmered in water for an extended amount of time, a pot or saucepan made of stainless steel is the most suitable vessel for heating the combination. In addition, a cheesecloth or a filter with a fine mesh is required to remove the herbs before they are consumed.

Proper labeling is necessary when recognizing herbs and herbal preparations and keeping track of their expiration dates. Labeling supplies are essential. Due to their ability to tolerate moisture and the ease with which they may be removed or replaced, waterproof labels or adhesive stickers are an excellent choice for identifying glass jars and bottles. Furthermore, a permanent marker or label printer can be utilized to write or print specific information regarding the herb. This information may include the herb's common name, Latin name, date of harvest, and any further instructions or precautions that may be considered necessary.

Accessories for Storage: If you want to make the most of the space on your shelves and improve your organization, you should consider purchasing storage accessories like spice racks, shelf organizers, and drawer dividers. When you are producing herbal medicines or cooking with herbs, these accessories can help you keep your herbs and herbal supplies neatly organized and easily accessible, making it easier for you to find what you need.

When it comes to effectively preparing and storing herbs and herbal treatments, it is necessary to have the appropriate instruments and supplies at your disposal. This includes harvesting instruments, drying equipment, storage containers, grinding and mixing equipment, tincture supplies, infusion and decoction equipment, labeling supplies, and storage accessories. All these things are necessary to keep the quality and potency of herbs and herbal products intact. You can be assured that your herbs will remain valid and fresh for use in culinary recipes, herbal treatments, and natural healthcare practices if you invest in high-quality equipment and appropriate storage methods.

Recipes for Herbal Remedies Step-by-step guides for common preparations

Herbal remedy recipes provide a safe, all-natural approach to treat various illnesses and enhance general health. Herbal preparations, which range from calming teas to therapeutic salves, can be customized to fit specific requirements and tastes. Here, we'll look at how-to manuals for popular herbal cures, which include thorough directions for making and applying these all-natural remedies.

One of the most accessible and adaptable methods to take advantage of the health benefits of herbs is to make herbal teas. Bring water to a boil in a pot or kettle before preparing a herbal tea. Gather the herbs you choose and measure the right amount for your recipe in the interim. Transfer the herbs to a mug or teapot and cover with boiling water. Depending on how strong and flavorful you want your herbs to be, steep them in the pot or mug for 5 to 10 minutes. Enjoy the tea hot or cold after straining it to remove the herbs. Popular tea ingredients include peppermint for digestion, ginger for immunity, and chamomile for relaxation.

To extract more robust characteristics, herbs are steeped in hot water for a more extended period, much like in herbal tea. The first step in creating a herbal infusion is to put the appropriate herbs in a teapot or glass container. Pour the slightly boiled water over the herbs, submerging them well. If covered and left in the jar or teapot, the herbs should simmer for at least four hours or overnight for a more potent infusion. After the herbs have been steeped, drain them and pour the liquid into a sanitized container to store it. Drinking infusions as a beverage or applying them topically as a compress or rinse helps treat many skin ailments.

Herbal Tincture: Herbs steeped in glycerin or alcohol yield concentrated herbal tinctures. To maximize surface area, finely chop or ground the desired herbs before making a herbal tincture. Make sure the liquid completely covers the herbs by placing them in a glass jar and covering them with alcohol or glycerin. To combine the contents, firmly seal the container and shake it well. To guarantee complete extraction, keep the jar in a cool, dark place for at least four to six weeks and shake it occasionally. After soaking the mixture, strain it using cheesecloth or a fine-mesh strainer to extract the herbs. Then, pour the tincture into dark glass bottles to preserve it. Tinctures can be applied locally to treat various skin disorders or eaten orally by diluting them in juice or water.

Herbal salves are topical ointments created by mixing herbs with beeswax for consistency and infusing them into a carrier oil. First, choose the desired herbs and chop or grind them finely before making an herbal salve. Put the herbs in a heat-resistant container and drizzle some carrier oil—like coconut or olive oil—over them. Using a double boiler or a heatproof dish placed over a saucepan of simmering water, slowly heat the mixture, stirring from time to time, until the oil is infused with the flavor of the herbs. After straining the oil through cheesecloth or a fine-mesh filter to remove the herbs, put the heated crude back on the burner and thicken it with beeswax. When the beeswax has melted, transfer the liquid into sanitized jars or tins and let it cool before capping the containers. The topical application of herbal salves helps relieve minor skin irritations, wounds, burns, and insect bites.

Indulging in an opulent herbal bath soak is a delightful method to de-stress and experience the health benefits of herbs. First, pick your preferred herbs and put them in a large cheesecloth pouch or muslin bag to make an herbal bath soak. As you fill the tub, hang the pouch from the bathtub faucet and run hot water over it. Before hopping in, let the herbs steep in the water for ten to fifteen minutes at the very least. To improve the experience, add extra components like essential oils for aromatherapy or Epsom salts for muscle relaxation. Herbal bath soaks can ease tense muscles, encourage relaxation, and aid in cleansing.

To sum up, there are many ways to use the therapeutic potential of plants, including through the creation of herbal remedy recipes. There is a herbal preparation to meet your needs, whether you want to improve your overall health or address specific health issues. You can enjoy the many advantages of herbal medicine and make your natural treatments at home by following these easy-to-follow instructions.

CHAPTER VI

Integrating Herbal Antibiotics into Daily Life

Preventative Use of Herbs

Herbal medicine, as a preventative, embraces a holistic approach to health and wellness, emphasizing balance and bolstering the body's innate defenses to fend off disease and extend life. Many civilizations have long used herbal treatments to defend themselves against illness and preserve good health. As more individuals look for natural alternatives to traditional therapy and try to be proactive with their health, the preventative use of herbs is becoming increasingly popular.

The immune system's potential to be strengthened by herbs is one of the advantages of utilizing them preventatively. Numerous herbs have immuno-modulating qualities that assist in controlling the body's immune response and improve its defenses against infections and viruses. Due to their well-known immune-stimulating properties, herbs like echinacea, astragalus, and elderberry are excellent friends in winter or when people are more prone to illness. You can boost your immunity and lower your disease risk by using these herbs in your daily routine, whether as supplements, tinctures, or teas.

Herbs are essential for boosting general energy well-being and immunological function. Numerous herbs have high concentrations of nutrients, minerals, antioxidants, and other bioactive substances that support and nourish the body's systems. Herbs with tonic qualities and high nutrient content, such as dandelion, alfalfa, and nettle, are suitable for general health and energy. By incorporating these herbs into your diet or taking them as supplements, you can ensure your body gets the vital nutrients it needs to function at its best and remain resilient to stressors.

Herbs are also frequently utilized as a prophylactic measure to assist particular bodily systems and organs. Herbs that nourish the liver, such as dandelion root and milk thistle, are well known for their ability to cleanse and enhance liver function. Similarly, spices like garlic and hawthorn improve average circulation, cholesterol levels, and blood pressure, which are suitable for cardiovascular health. Using these herbs in your wellness routine can boost the health of particular organs and systems and lower your chance of developing chronic illnesses over time.

The capacity of herbs to promote mental and emotional health is another benefit of using them as a preventative measure. Numerous plants have nervine and adaptogenic qualities that boost cognitive function, ease stress, and encourage relaxation. Herbs that help soothe the nervous system and increase stress tolerance include ashwagandha, holy basil, and lemon balm. Using teas, tinctures, or aromatherapy, you can boost your mental and emotional well-being and improve your general quality of life by adding these herbs to your daily routine.

In conclusion, employing herbs as a preventative measure provides a comprehensive, natural approach to health and wellness that emphasizes preserving equilibrium and assisting the body's natural healing processes. You may fortify your immune system, encourage vitality, support organ health, and improve mental and emotional well-being by adding immune-boosting herbs, nutrient-dense tonics, organ-specific supports, and nervine adaptogens to your daily routine. Herbs can contribute significantly to the prevention of disease and the promotion of optimum health for many years to come, whether utilized as teas, tinctures, supplements, or culinary items.

Strengthening the immune system

Maintaining health and resistance to infections and illnesses requires strengthening the immune system. The immune system is a complex network of cells, tissues, and organs that fights bacteria, viruses, and fungi. It protects the body, but many things can impair it, making people more susceptible to illness. Fortunately, herbs and other natural methods can boost the immune system and prevent illnesses.

An effective strategy to boost immunity is through appropriate eating. A diet rich in vitamins, minerals, antioxidants, and other nutrients builds a robust immune system. Certain herbs are immune-boosting, making them essential supplements to a healthy diet. Echinacea is known for stimulating white blood cell formation, which fights infections. Elderberry, rich in flavonoids and anthocyanins, inhibits viral multiplication and shortens colds and flu.

Maintaining a robust immune system requires good nutrition and stress management. Chronic stress lowers immune function, rendering people more prone to infections. Luckily, many herbs are adaptogenic, helping the body adapt to stress and preserve equilibrium. Ashwagandha, holy basil, and reishi mushrooms are valued for their stress-modulating, cortisol-lowering, and resilience-boosting properties. Utilizing adaptogenic herbs in teas, tinctures, or supplements might reduce stress's adverse effects on the immune system and improve general health.

To support immune function, promote a healthy lifestyle through frequent exercise, sleep, and hygiene. Exercise increases circulation, reduces inflammation, and boosts immune cell production, helping the body fight illnesses. Quality sleep helps the body repair and regenerate cells, optimize immunological function, and produce cytokines, which govern the immune response. Avoiding direct contact with sick people, washing hands, and keeping surfaces clean reduces the risk of pathogen exposure and diseases.

Finally, including immune-supportive herbs in your wellness routine can boost immunity. Garlic, astragalus, and medicinal mushrooms like shiitake and maitake, along with echinacea and elderberry, boost immune response and infection resistance. These herbs contain bioactive components like allicin, polysaccharides, and beta-glucans that boost immune cell activation and pathogen defense. Adding these herbs to your diet or taking supplements can boost your immune system and minimize disease.

Finally, boosting the immune system is crucial for good health and disease resistance. A comprehensive strategy that combines good nutrition, stress management, healthy lifestyle choices, and immune-supportive herbs can boost immunity and minimize sickness. Herbal teas, tinctures, and supplements boost immunity and well-being.

Travel kit essentials

While traveling can be a thrilling and rewarding experience, it's essential to be ready for everything that might come up. A well-equipped travel kit guarantees you will have all you require to remain secure, comfortable, and healthy while traveling. To ensure a seamless and pleasurable journey, your travel kit should always contain a few necessities, regardless of whether you're going on a quick weekend vacation or a lengthy expedition.

First and foremost, when traveling, personal hygiene supplies are necessary to keep oneself clean and avoid getting sick. Travel-sized bottles of body wash, shampoo, conditioner, toothbrush, toothpaste, and floss are some of these supplies. Pack tissues, hand sanitizer, and antibacterial wipes to keep hands hygienic and free of germs, mainly when access to soap and water is scarce. Using lip balm and sunscreen with SPF protection is also essential to protect your skin from UV rays outside.

Your travel kit should also contain medical supplies for minor health problems while away from home. Keep an over-the-counter medicine kit with bandages, adhesive tape, antiseptic wipes, and other supplies for treating pain, fever, and stomach distress. In an emergency, it's a good idea to have a copy of your prescriptions and medical history with you, along with any prescription drugs you require. If you visit places where motion sickness, allergies, or insect bites are common, consider packing motion sickness medication, antihistamines, and insect repellent.

Apart from essential personal care and medical supplies, including valuable products to improve your ease and comfort while traveling is crucial. These could include a reusable water bottle to stay hydrated during your trip, earplugs and an eye mask for peaceful sleep in loud or highly lit locations, and a travel cushion and blanket for lengthy bus or airplane travel. While a travel adapter guarantees that you may plug in and recharge your gadgets in multiple countries, a portable phone charger or power bank is also helpful for keeping your electronic devices on the go.

In addition, remember to take the necessary paperwork and things for your trip to ensure a hassle-free and easy journey. These could consist of copies of vital documents, including your itinerary, hotel bookings, and emergency contacts, as well as your passport, driver's license, and information on your trip insurance. For day travels or sightseeing excursions, a lightweight backpack or daypack helps transport necessities, and a money belt or neck pouch offers a covert and safe method to carry valuables like cash, credit cards, and travel documents.

To sum up, having a fully packed travel kit is crucial to guaranteeing a relaxing, risk-free, and delightful trip. Your travel kit should contain personal hygiene products, medical supplies, valuable accessories, and essential documents to prepare you for everything that might arise while traveling. Whether you're traveling domestically or abroad, for work or pleasure, having the correct necessities on hand can make all the difference in the success of your trip.

Tips for staying healthy on the go

Maintaining your health when traveling is crucial to a pleasurable and stress-free trip. Traveling for business, pleasure, or a weekend break should all revolve around keeping your health and well-being in mind. Fortunately, no matter where your travels take you, you can maintain your health and vitality while on the road with a few easy methods and recommendations.

Drink plenty of water first and foremost while you travel. Dehydration during travel, mainly by air or in a hot environment, can result in headaches, exhaustion, and other health problems. Aim to stay hydrated during the day by packing a reusable water bottle and consuming plenty of water, herbal teas, and electrolyte-rich drinks. Steer clear of excessive alcohol or caffeine intake since they can exacerbate dehydration. Carry hydrating snacks like fresh fruits and vegetables to maintain hydration levels and give necessary nutrients while running.

Sustaining general health and well-being when traveling also requires eating a balanced diet. While traveling, eating unhealthy snacks or fast food can be tempting, but choosing thoughtful food choices will keep you feeling nourished and energized the entire time. Seek out eateries or supermarkets that provide wholesome selections like salads, grilled meats, and whole grains. Pack healthy snacks such as dried fruits, granola bars, nuts, and seeds to relieve hunger between meals. In addition, think about packing an insulated bag or small cooler to store perishable goods and maintain their freshness while you're on the road.

To maintain your physical and emotional well-being when on the go, prioritize rest and relaxation in addition to eating healthfully and drinking plenty of water. Traveling can be emotionally and physically exhausting, so paying attention to your body's needs and taking breaks when necessary to rejuvenate is important. Whether you're traveling long distances by car, airline, or train, take breaks to stretch your legs, get some fresh air, and release any tension in your muscles. During your trip, try relaxation exercises like deep breathing, meditation, or light stretching to help you decompress and feel more at ease.

Prioritize personal hygiene to stop the spread of germs and lower your chance of getting sick when traveling. Use hand sanitizer when there aren't any handwashing facilities, and wash your hands often with soap and water, especially before eating or touching your face. Refrain from using unwashed hands to touch your mouth, nose, eyes, or face since this can spread bacteria and raise your risk of infection. Always have antibacterial hand gel or disinfectant wipes to clean surfaces like tray tables, armrests, and door handles in public areas.

Finally, remember to maintain your activity level and include physical activity in your holiday plans to promote general health and well-being. Take a nature stroll or a picturesque hike, explore your area on foot or by bike, or partake in an outdoor adventure activity or fitness class. Being physically active is crucial for maintaining good health when on the go because it keeps muscles and the heart healthy, improves mood, and lowers stress levels.

In summary, maintaining good health when traveling necessitates a proactive attitude to rest, food, hydration, cleanliness, and physical activity. No matter where your travels take you, you may have a secure, comfortable, and gratifying trip by putting five critical areas of health and well-being first. Whether you're traveling domestically or abroad, for work or pleasure, taking care of yourself while traveling will help guarantee that you return home feeling revitalized and eager for your next adventure.

Combining Herbs with Modern Medicine

Herbs and modern medicine are being used together as individuals attempt to combine the benefits of each. Herbal therapy supports health and well-being naturally and holistically, unlike contemporary medicine, which treats acute and chronic diseases. Integrating herbs with modern medication can improve health when done carefully and under medical supervision.

Combining herbs with contemporary medication may improve treatment outcomes due to synergistic effects. Many botanicals include bioactive components that enhance pharmaceutical drugs, improving symptom alleviation and illness management. Some herbs improve medicine absorption and efficacy, while others reduce side effects or improve treatment response. Integrating herbs into a holistic treatment plan allows doctors to personalize interventions to each patient's requirements and preferences, increasing therapeutic outcomes and quality of life.

Herbs can also help the body's natural healing processes and promote well-being, complementing modern treatment. Instead of treating symptoms or suppressing disease, herbal medicine addresses fundamental imbalances and supports the body's natural healing process. Echinacea, garlic, and ginger enhance immunity and help the body fight illnesses and stress. Chamomile, lavender, and valerian calm and relax, supporting mental health and well-being.

Herbal treatments can also enable individuals to manage their health and well-being, boosting autonomy and self-efficacy. Many people are drawn to herbal therapy because of its natural and holistic approach to health, which emphasizes nutrition, stress management, physical activity, and herbal medicines. Herbs can help patients stay healthy and prevent illness, complementing modern therapy and sometimes lowering the pharmaceutical need.

However, integrating herbs with contemporary medicine requires caution and alertness due to potential hazards and interactions. Herbs are generally safe when used properly, although they can interact with pharmaceuticals and may not be suitable for everyone, especially pregnant or breastfeeding women. Before adding herbs to their treatment plan, patients should speak with doctors, pharmacists, or licensed herbalists to ensure safety and efficacy.

Finally, mixing herbs with contemporary medicine provides a holistic approach to healthcare that can improve treatment outcomes, promote well-being, and empower individuals to manage their health. Patients can maximize therapeutic outcomes, quality of life, and synergy between herbal and pharmaceutical therapies by including herbs in a comprehensive treatment plan under the supervision of experienced healthcare professionals. Herbs and modern medicine can transform health and wellness in the 21st century if patients and doctors work together.

How to work with healthcare providers

Effective communication with healthcare providers is vital for personalized, comprehensive care that matches your health requirements and goals. Collaborating with your healthcare team is essential to improving your health, whether treating a specific ailment, managing chronic health conditions, or optimizing your overall well-being how to advocate for your health and get the most excellent care with healthcare providers.

Communicating with healthcare providers comes first. Share your health issues, symptoms, medical history, medications, supplements, and alternative therapies. Giving your healthcare team accurate and precise information helps them make informed decisions and customize treatment programs. Request clarity about your diagnosis, treatment options, and prognosis. Understanding your health status and reasons for recommended treatments empowers you to engage in your care and make educated health decisions actively.

Proactively advocate for your health and priorities.

Remember that you are the expert on your body and have the right to participate in care decisions. Communicate your treatment objectives and preferences to your healthcare team and work together to create a plan that meets your needs. If you believe your concerns need to be addressed or have questions or doubts about a planned treatment plan, speak out. Your doctors should respect your autonomy and work with you to create a personalized strategy.

Establish trust and respect with your healthcare staff to encourage collaboration. Recognize that healthcare practitioners are experts and provide vital information. Respect and trust others and listen to their advice. Expect to be treated with dignity and respect, and speak out if you feel your issues are not being addressed or are discriminated against. A good relationship with your healthcare team promotes open communication, trust, and a shared health goal.

Take charge of your health by following treatment, medication, and lifestyle adjustments. Schedule visits, have testing, and follow your doctor's orders. Keep note of your symptoms, progress, and health changes, and inform your doctors at follow-up appointments. Take responsibility for your health and actively participate in your care to increase treatment efficacy, health outcomes, and quality of life.

In conclusion, effective healthcare-provider collaboration is vital for optimal health outcomes and tailored care that fits your needs and aspirations. Open communication, advocating for your health, creating trust and mutual respect, and actively managing your health can help you collaborate with your healthcare team to get the most outstanding results. Remember that you are the best advocate for your health, and by actively participating in your care, you can take charge and live your best life.

CHAPTER VII

Advanced Topics in Herbal Antibiotics

Herbal Synergies and Combinations

Combining different herbs to maximize their therapeutic effects and produce a more all-encompassing and well-rounded approach to health and wellness is known as herbal synergies and combinations. Herbalists and healers have known for ages that some herbs have complementary qualities that, when combined, work synergistically to produce more therapeutic benefit and efficacy than when used alone. Herbal synergies and combinations can address various health conditions and promote general well-being by carefully choosing and mixing herbs based on their distinct qualities and activities.

The capacity of herbal synergies and combinations to target several facets of health and treat intricate medical disorders is one of their main benefits. Numerous herbs have various pharmacological characteristics, such as adaptogenic, antioxidant, antibacterial, and anti-inflammatory actions. Herbalists can formulate remedies that address specific health issues from several perspectives by mixing plants with complimentary effects, offering a more thorough and efficient treatment. For instance, combining turmeric, ginger, and boswellia can help with arthritis pain and inflammation while promoting healthy digestion and general well-being.

Moreover, the synergies and combinations of herbs can improve the absorption and bioavailability of active ingredients, resulting in increased therapeutic efficacy. Certain chemicals found in herbs can improve the body's ability to absorb other nutrients or move them across cell membranes, making them more bioavailable and effective. For instance, the active ingredient in turmeric, curcumin, can be absorbed up to 2,000% more readily when piperine, a component found in black pepper, is added. Herbalists can increase the absorption of curcumin and strengthen its anti-inflammatory and antioxidant properties by mixing it with black pepper.

Additionally, when utilizing specific herbs, herbal synergies and combinations might assist in reducing the possibility of adverse effects and increase tolerance. Certain plants have solid and stimulating properties that, when taken by themselves, may be overpowering or overly strong, causing uncomfortable side effects. Herbalists can reduce the possibility of adverse effects and create formulations well-tolerated by a wider variety of people by mixing these plants with softer or more balanced herbs. For instance, balancing the impact of stimulating herbs like rhodiola or ginseng with relaxing herbs like chamomile or lemon balm might lower the risk of agitation or overstimulation.

Herbal synergies and combinations can also tailor therapies to patients' requirements and preferences. Due to variances in metabolism, constitution, and state of health, no two persons are alike; therefore, what suits one may not suit another. Herbalists can customize remedies to target specific health issues and enhance general well-being by combining herbs according to patient requirements and preferences. For instance, a combination of nervine herbs like passionflower and skullcap and adaptogenic herbs like ashwagandha and holy basil may help stressed and anxious people by supporting relaxation and fostering emotional equilibrium.

In conclusion, herbal synergies and combinations offer a comprehensive and individualized approach to health and wellness by using the complementary qualities of several herbs to increase therapeutic efficacy, improve tolerance, and treat complicated health concerns. Herbalists can design formulations that attack certain health conditions from several aspects, offering a more comprehensive and successful approach to treatment by carefully choosing and mixing herbs based on their distinct properties and effects. Herbal synergies and combinations provide a flexible and effective tool for naturally boosting health and well-being, whether employed to improve bioavailability, reduce side effects, or customize treatments.

Combining herbs for enhanced effect

Combining herbs for maximum impact has its roots in the extensive history of herbal medicine, which maximizes the therapeutic effects of several plants by utilizing their synergistic interactions. Herbalists and healers have known for ages that some plants contain contrasting qualities that can have more powerful and all-encompassing effects than when taken separately. By carefully selecting and mixing herbs based on their distinct properties and effects, herbalists can design formulations that attack specific health conditions from various sides, providing a more holistic and effective approach to health and wellness.

The capacity to target complicated health concerns and address numerous elements of health is one of the main benefits of combining herbs for greater efficacy. Numerous herbs have various bioactive substances, each with unique pharmacological characteristics and effects. Herbalists can produce formulations that target the root causes of health concerns and support harmony and balance inside the body by mixing herbs with complementary activities. For instance, a more thorough and all-encompassing approach to treatment may be taken by combining herbs like turmeric, ginger, and black pepper to target inflammation, pain, and digestive problems all at once.

Moreover, mixing herbs to maximize their effects might increase the active components' bioavailability and absorption, which boosts their medicinal efficacy. Certain herbs have substances that improve other nutrients' absorption or help them pass through cell membranes, increasing their bioavailability and potency in the body. For instance, the active ingredient in turmeric, curcumin, can be absorbed up to 2,000% more readily when piperine, a component found in black pepper, is added. Herbalists can increase the absorption of curcumin and strengthen its anti-inflammatory and antioxidant properties by mixing it with black pepper.

Additionally, combining several herbs for a more significant effect can reduce the possibility of adverse effects and increase the acceptability of some herbs. Certain plants have solid and stimulating properties that, when taken by themselves, may be overpowering or overly strong, causing uncomfortable side effects. Herbalists can reduce the possibility of adverse effects and create formulations well-tolerated by a wider variety of people by mixing these plants with softer or more balanced herbs. For instance, balancing the impact of stimulating herbs like rhodiola or ginseng with relaxing herbs like chamomile or lemon balm might help lower the risk of agitation or overstimulation.

Herbalists can also more easily and specifically customize herbal formulations by combining herbs for optimal impact. This enables them to create customized medicines catering to each patient's needs and preferences. Due to variances in metabolism, constitution, and state of health, no two persons are alike; therefore, what suits one may not suit another. Herbalists can build individualized remedies that target specific health issues and promote general well-being by combining herbs according to each person's requirements and preferences. Combining herbs to maximize their effects can be used to improve bioavailability, reduce adverse effects, or customize treatments. It's a flexible and effective way to support health and wellness organically.

Recipes and formulations

The foundation of herbal medicine consists of recipes and formulations that offer a valuable and efficient means of utilizing plants' curative abilities for various medical issues. Herbal preparations, which can be used topically to support health and well-being, are made by carefully choosing and combining herbs with other components like oils, honey, or alcohol. These concoctions come in a variety of forms, each customized to suit individual requirements and tastes, including teas, tinctures, salves, poultices, and capsules.

One of their main advantages is the capacity of recipes and formulations to be customized to meet specific needs and tastes. Herbalists can consider a person's specific health concerns, constitution, and lifestyle when creating custom formulations, which enables a personalized approach to health and wellness. Herbal formulas are a great way to match each person's specific needs, offering focused support and comfort for acute ailments like colds and flu and chronic conditions like arthritis and digestive disorders.

In addition, recipes and formulations provide a comprehensive approach to wellness and health by addressing the root causes of illnesses and fostering harmony and balance inside the body. A wide range of bioactive chemicals, each with unique pharmacological characteristics and activities, are present in many herbs. Herbalists can produce formulations that address several facets of health and offer all-encompassing support for the body's inherent healing processes by mixing herbs with complementary effects. For instance, a blend intended to assist digestive well-being can incorporate herbs such as peppermint, fennel, and ginger, each of which has unique advantages for easing discomfort and aiding digestion.

Furthermore, formulations and recipes make it possible to create herbal medicines that are user-friendly and convenient, which makes it simpler for people to include herbal medicine in their regular routines. When people make herbal remedies at home, they can control the quality and potency of the ingredients more closely, guaranteeing that they get the full therapeutic effects of the herbs. Herbal recipes can be easy to follow and accessible to individuals of all skill levels, whether you're making a batch of tea to drink throughout the day or a soothing salve to apply to painful muscles.

Herbalists can also use recipes and formulations for experimentation and creativity, testing out novel combinations of herbs and ingredients to treat new health issues or adjust to shifting climates and seasons. With so many different spices and other natural ingredients, countless options exist for making distinctive and potent mixtures. Herbalists can customize treatments to match the changing requirements of people and communities, whether creating novel new formulations based on the most recent scientific research or adhering to traditional formulas handed down through the decades.

To sum up, formulas and recipes are crucial tools in herbal medicine since they provide a valuable and efficient means of utilizing plants' curative abilities for various medical issues. Herbal formulas can be customized to fit individuals' unique needs and preferences, offering focused support and relief for both acute and chronic diseases. Recipes and formulations, with their adaptability, ease, and versatility, enable people to naturally take charge of their health and well-being, utilizing the power of plants to support health and vitality for both themselves and their communities.

Cultivating Your Own Medicinal Herbs

Grow medicinal herbs in your backyard for a satisfying and uplifting experience. Growing medical plants for personal use, making herbal treatments, or connecting with nature can improve physical and mental health. Cultivating herbs yourself guarantees the freshest and most potent herbs. Connecting yourself to plants and nature and cultivating therapeutic herbs also helps you appreciate, respect, and steward the environment and its resources.

Growing your medical herbs allows you to access many plants that may not be available in supermarkets or markets. Many medicinal herbs are climate-specific and hard to find commercially. By cultivating them yourself, you can guarantee a regular supply of fresh, powerful herbs for personal use or herbal treatments. Growing medical herbs lets you try numerous types and species to find the ones that suit your needs.

Growing medicinal herbs sustainably promotes biodiversity and conservation. Many therapeutic herbs are threatened by overharvesting, habitat loss, and other environmental factors. Planting these herbs can safeguard endangered species and plant genetic variety. Organic and regenerative herb agriculture reduces hazardous chemicals and pesticides, improving soil and ecosystem health.

Growing your medicinal herbs helps you understand herbal medicine and plant healing. You'll learn about herbs' therapeutic characteristics, growth habits, and ideal growing circumstances while you care for them. This hands-on experience strengthens your connection to plants and improves your capacity to employ them as health cures. Cultivating medical herbs helps herbalists learn and improve, whether making teas and tinctures or drying and preserving them.

Besides their practical and therapeutic benefits, growing medicinal herbs has mental and emotional benefits. Gardening is a relaxing way to connect with nature and find peace in its rhythms. Gardening reduces stress, anxiety, and sadness, boosts mood, and gives people a feeling of purpose. Growing medicinal herbs can bring joy, inspiration, and healing to your body and soul, whether you tend to them, harvest them, or just enjoy their aroma and beauty.

Finally, growing therapeutic herbs is a beautiful and enlightening experience that promotes physical, mental, and emotional health. By cultivating them yourself, you can guarantee the freshest and most potent herbs. You may also encourage biodiversity and conservation, connect with nature, and grow therapeutic herbs sustainably. Growing medical herbs is a great way to nourish your body, mind, and soul while connecting with the land and its richness, whether making herbal remedies, studying plant healing, or just enjoying gardening.

Gardening tips and techniques

Growing their own food, creating beautiful outdoor places, and connecting with nature are all possible through gardening, which is a gratifying and enjoyable hobby. Several strategies and tactics can help you succeed in your undertakings and make the most of your gardening efforts, regardless of your expertise level.

Selecting the ideal site for your garden should be your top priority. Because most plants need at least six to eight hours of sunshine to grow, please choose a location that receives plenty throughout the day. Additionally, make sure the area has well-drained soil to avoid waterlogging and root rot. When deciding where to put your garden, take accessibility, wind exposure, and closeness to water sources into account.

After deciding on a spot, you need to prepare the soil. A thriving garden is built on healthy soil, which gives plants the vital nutrients, water, and oxygen they need. To enhance drainage and aeration, start by clearing the area of any weeds, rocks, or debris. Then, use a shovel or garden fork to loosen the soil. To increase the soil's fertility and texture, add organic matter, such as compost, aged manure, or leaf mold.

When designing your garden's structure, consider elements like crop rotation, companion planting, and plant spacing to optimize yields and reduce pest and disease issues. Taller plants, including maize, tomatoes, and peppers, should be planted at the back of the garden so they won't shade out shorter plants. Planting companion crops, which group similar crops together to ward off pests or promote growth, might also be advantageous. For instance, planting marigolds next to tomatoes helps deter nematodes and other pests.

Another essential component of a successful garden is watering. Most plants need regular hydration, especially in hot weather or during dry spells. Make sure to water your garden thoroughly and deeply so that the soil is equally moist but not overly wet. To ensure that water reaches the roots of plants, use a drip irrigation system or soaker hose rather than overhead watering, which can encourage the spread of fungal infections.

Proper mulching can help your garden retain moisture, discourage weed growth, and control soil temperature, in addition to watering. To assist in retaining moisture and enhance the health of the soil surrounding your plants, spread a layer of organic mulch, such as wood chips, straw, or crushed leaves. In addition, mulching creates a home for helpful microbes and insects that improve soil fertility and plant health.

Last but not least, remember to routinely check your garden for indications of pests, illnesses, or nutritional shortages. It's imperative to identify issues early on and take action to stop them from getting worse and harming your plants extensively. Look out for common garden pests like slugs, aphids, and caterpillars. To eliminate them, use organic methods like handpicking, insecticidal soap, or biological remedies.

To sum up, gardening is a fulfilling and pleasurable hobby with several advantages for mental, emotional, and physical health. By implementing the strategies and recommendations listed below, you can have a flourishing garden that gives you year-round access to fresh, healthful produce and a lovely outside area. There's always something new to learn and uncover in the garden, regardless of your level of gardening expertise. Thus, put on some gloves, get your hands dirty, and allow the delight of gardening to enhance your existence!

Best herbs to grow at home

Growing a variety of savory and aromatic herbs in your garden or windowsill is fun and gratifying. Many herbs can thrive in various growing situations and are suitable for home production. These are the most excellent herbs to grow at home, from culinary to medicinal.

Basil is a popular plant for home production due to its flavor and culinary flexibility. Basil grows well from seed or transplants in warm, sunny, well-drained soil. Fresh basil leaves provide flavor to salads, pasta, and sauces, and its fragrant foliage enhances herb gardens and containers.

Another cooking essential that grows nicely at home is parsley, which has a vibrant flavor and nutritional value. Parsley grows well in deep, wet soil from seed or transplant in partial shade. Fresh parsley leaves provide color to garden beds and containers and are adaptable in soups, stews, salads, and sauces.

Chives, with their mild onion flavor and easy growth, are another great home gardener alternative. They grow best in sunny, well-drained soil from seed or transplant. The plant's exquisite lavender blossoms are edible and make a lovely garnish, while its slender, grass-like leaves can be picked fresh and used to make omelets, salads, and baked potatoes.

With its intense flavor and fragrant foliage, Rosemary is famous for home growing. Full sun and well-drained soil are ideal for increasing rosemary from seed, cuttings, or transplants. Rosemary leaves offer roasted meats, vegetables, and bread taste, and its woody stems look great in herb gardens and containers.

Another popular herb that proliferates at home is thyme, its earthy flavor and aromatic leaf. Thyme grows from seed or transplants in whole light and well-drained soil. The plant's low growth makes it great for edging garden beds or filling gaps in herb gardens and containers, and fresh thyme leaves give depth to soups, stews, sauces, and marinades.

In addition to culinary herbs, several medicinal herbs can be grown at home to improve health. Lavender, which calms and soothes, can be grown from seed or transplants in sunny, well-drained soil. Fresh lavender blooms produce herbal drinks, sachets, and bath treatments, while aromatic foliage beautifies garden beds and containers.

Other popular medical herbs that are easy to produce include peppermint, which has a pleasant taste and digestive advantages. Peppermint grows from seed or transplants in moist, well-drained soil in moderate shade. Fresh peppermint leaves create herbal drinks, infused oils, and tinctures, and the plant's spreading tendency makes it a good ground cover for gloomy gardens.

In conclusion, growing herbs in your garden or windowsill is a fun and gratifying way to develop a variety of delectable and aromatic plants. Many culinary and medicinal herbs can be grown at home and thrive in a range of situations. Roll up your sleeves, get dirty, and enjoy herb gardening!

CHAPTER VIII

Herbal Antibiotics for Children and Pets

Special Considerations for Children

Extra measures must be taken to guarantee the safety and efficacy of herbal treatments for children. While many herbs provide health benefits for children, taking caution and care while using them is essential because children may be more vulnerable to some herb effects and may have specific health needs. When utilizing herbal medicines for children, there are a few critical things to remember.

First and foremost, before administering herbal treatments to children—especially newborns, toddlers, and young children—it is imperative to speak with a licensed healthcare professional. Since their bodies are still developing, children's physiologies may differ significantly from adults', impacting how they metabolize and react to herbal therapies. A pediatric herbal medicine specialist can offer tailored suggestions based on the child's age, weight, overall health, and any underlying medical issues.

Furthermore, it's critical to find safe, mild medicines for kids that are age—and developmentally appropriate and easy to tolerate. Certain herbs might be excessively potent or stimulating for young children, and others might have negative effects or conflict with prescription drugs. Before administering any herb, it is imperative to conduct a comprehensive investigation of its safety profile and suitability for use with children.

It's also critical to employ the proper dosages and administration techniques to guarantee the safety and efficacy of herbal treatments when given to children. Children's dosages vary according to their age, weight, and health status and are often lower than those for adults. It's crucial to precisely administer herbal treatments to children by using measurement tools like syringes or droppers and to adhere to dosage recommendations given by a licensed healthcare professional.

Furthermore, it's critical to watch out for any negative responses or side effects while using herbal medicines on kids and to stop using them right once if they do. Children may be more susceptible to the effects of herbs, and particular cures may cause allergic responses, unsettled stomachs, or other adverse side effects. It is imperative to commence with minimal dosages and progressively raise as necessary while constantly observing the child's reaction to the treatment.

Additionally, it's critical to teach kids about the responsible and safe use of herbal remedies and urge them to consult adults with any queries about using herbs. When taking herbal treatments, children should know the significance of correct dosage, administration, and monitoring for adverse effects. They should also always seek adult supervision when using herbs, mainly if young or inexperienced.

In conclusion, even though children's health can benefit from herbal therapies, extra care and attention must be given to assure their efficacy and safety. When using herbal remedies for children, it's essential to follow specific guidelines, such as speaking with a licensed healthcare professional, selecting gentle and safe remedies, utilizing the proper dosages and administration techniques, keeping an eye out for side effects, and teaching kids about the responsible and safe use of herbs. Parents and other caregivers can naturally and safely support their children's health and well-being by using herbal remedies with caution and attention.

Dosage adjustments

Making necessary dosage changes is essential to administering herbal treatments safely and successfully, particularly when addressing individual variations in tolerance levels, age, weight, and health state. Herbal medicines have many health advantages, but dosages should be customized to each person's unique needs to achieve the best outcomes and reduce the possibility of side effects.

The patient's age is one of the most essential variables when adjusting the dosage. Different metabolic rates, body weights, and physiological parameters may necessitate lesser dosages of herbal treatments in children, infants, and elderly adults than in healthy adults. Infants and young children can be more susceptible to the effects of herbs; therefore, in order to prevent negative responses, lower, more diluted doses may be necessary.

Additionally, weight may need to be taken into account when adjusting dosages because larger people could need higher doses to get the appropriate therapeutic effect. Furthermore, a person's health status and any underlying medical disorders may require dosage adjustments. When utilizing herbal medicines, people with weakened immune systems, long-term medical issues, or those taking medication may need to use smaller dosages or take extra care to prevent drug interactions or negative effects.

Furthermore, dosages need to be changed by each person's tolerance level and herbal remedy response. Some people are more susceptible to the effects of specific herbs, so they would need to take smaller doses to prevent negative effects like sleepiness, allergic reactions, or upset stomachs. It's crucial to begin with lesser dosages and increase them gradually as necessary while closely observing how the patient responds to the treatment.

Furthermore, depending on how the herbal treatment is prepared and its form, dosages could need to be changed. The body can absorb and process herbs differently depending on their potency and absorption rate. These variations can occur in tinctures, teas, capsules, or extracts. It's crucial to adhere to dose recommendations unique to the herbal remedy's form and preparation and to modify them according to personal requirements and preferences.

To sum up, dose adjustments are essential to utilizing herbal treatments safely and efficiently. They guarantee everyone receives the right herbs to fulfill their unique needs and health objectives. Doses can be adjusted to maximize therapeutic results and reduce the chance of side effects by considering the herbal remedy's form and preparation, age, weight, health status, and tolerance levels. To guarantee the safe and efficient use of herbal medicines, it is imperative to regularly monitor the patient's response to the remedy and consult with a certified healthcare practitioner before making any dosage adjustments.

Safe herbs for children

Safety is the most crucial factor when utilizing herbs with kids. Even though many herbs have therapeutic benefits for children's health, selecting herbs that are age- and developmentally appropriate, mild, and well-tolerated is essential. The following list of safe herbs for kids can be utilized to promote their overall health and well-being.

Because of its calming and soothing qualities, chamomile is one of the safest and most popular herbs for kids. It is a popular choice for parents looking for natural solutions for common childhood disorders. Chamomile can help relieve colic symptoms, discomfort associated with teething, and upset stomachs in newborns and early children. For older children, chamomile tea can be taken in tiny amounts or made and diluted for gentle pain relief. It also encourages relaxation and sound sleep.

Ginger is another safe plant for kids to treat nausea, indigestion, and upset stomachs. Grated ginger can be added to soups, smoothies, or baked goods to help soothe the stomach and promote digestion. It can also be brewed into a calming tea. Chewable tablets and ginger candies are also available for older kids who want a more convenient way to take them.

In addition, children can safely and effectively use peppermint to relieve upset stomach symptoms, such as bloating, gas, and pain in the abdomen. Older children can be given tiny amounts of peppermint tea to ease discomfort and support a healthy digestive system, or it can be made and diluted for newborns. Additionally, diluted peppermint oil can be administered topically to the chest or abdomen to help relieve lung congestion or upset stomach.

Furthermore, lemon balm is a safe herb for kids that can aid with anxiety reduction, relaxation promotion, and better sleep. Older children can be given tiny amounts of lemon balm tea or made and diluted for newborns to soothe anxiety, relieve tension, and encourage sound sleep. In addition, lemon balm can be added to bath water or applied directly as a mild herbal treatment for insect bites or skin irritations.

Furthermore, elderberry is a kid-safe and kid-effective herb that supports immune function and enhances respiratory health. Children often choose elderberry syrup or candies as a tasty and practical approach to strengthening immunity and preventing colds and the flu. Elderberries can be added to smoothies or porridge or made into tea for an additional immunological boost.

In conclusion, children can benefit from various safe herbs that can be used naturally to enhance their health and well-being. Herbs that are mild, easily tolerated, and suitable for kids of all ages include chamomile, ginger, peppermint, lemon balm, and elderberry. These safe herbs provide parents and caregivers with excellent alternatives for treating common kid diseases without harsh chemicals or pharmaceuticals, whether used to improve immune function, ease stomach disturbance, or encourage relaxation. As usual, to guarantee the safety and efficacy of herbs, it is imperative to speak with a licensed healthcare professional before administering them to children, particularly newborns or those with underlying medical issues.

Herbal Remedies for Pets

Pet owners have turned more and more to herbal medicines to manage their furry friends' health issues naturally and holistically instead of resorting to pharmaceuticals. Many herbs can safely and efficiently support the health and well-being of pets, from digestion problems and skin disorders to anxiety and joint discomfort. Animals may react to herbs differently than people do, so it's essential to use caution and care when using herbal medicines for pets. A closer look at herbal treatments for pets and how to utilize them to support health and vitality is provided here.

Supporting digestive health is one of the most popular applications for pet herbal treatments. Herbs that can relieve diarrhea or constipation, soothe irritated or inflamed digestive tissues, and support healthy gastrointestinal functions include marshmallow root, licorice, and slippery elm. These herbs can be added to pet food for simple intake or taken orally as teas, tinctures, or capsules.

Herbs can also promote the health of your pet's coat and skin. Calendula, chamomile, and lavender are examples of anti-inflammatory, antibacterial, and calming herbs that can help reduce the redness, irritation, and itching that come with skin diseases like dermatitis, allergies, and hot spots. These herbs can be added to pet baths for a calming and therapeutic effect or applied externally as infused oils, sprays, or salves.

Herbs can also be utilized to promote pet mobility and joint health. Herbs with anti-inflammatory and analgesic qualities, such as turmeric, ginger, and boswellia, can help lessen pain, swelling, and stiffness related to joint diseases such as hip dysplasia and arthritis. To reduce discomfort and increase movement, these herbs can be fed to pets or taken orally as supplements.

Herbs can also be utilized to promote pets' mental and behavioral well-being. Herbs with soothing and relaxing effects, like passionflower, skullcap, and valerian, can help pets feel less anxious, stressed, and tense. To aid relaxation and emotional balance, these herbs can be added to pet food or given orally as tinctures or teas.

Herbal treatments can be utilized in various ways to promote the health and well-being of dogs in addition to these typical ones. Milk thistle and dandelion are herbs that support liver and kidney health, while others, like astragalus and echinacea, help support pets' immune systems and shield them from infections and disease. Additionally, herbs like burdock and nettle can enhance pets' general health and vitality by offering crucial vitamins, minerals, and antioxidants.

Finally, using herbal medicines to enhance your pet's health and well-being is a natural and comprehensive strategy. Many herbs can be used safely and effectively to treat various health issues in pets, from anxiety and joint discomfort to skin disorders and digestive problems. Animals may react to herbs differently than people do, so it's essential to use caution and care when using herbal medicines for pets. Pet owners can ensure the safety and efficacy of their furry companions by choosing the best herbs and dosages in consultation with a certified veterinary herbalist or holistic veterinarian. Herbal treatments can be helpful in naturally boosting pets' health and vigor when used under proper direction and supervision.

Common ailments and treatments

Like us, our furry friends can suffer from common illnesses, and knowing these problems and how to manage them is essential to protecting our pets' health. Pets may have health problems that need quick notice and proper care, including respiratory infections, joint pain, and digestive and skin disorders. This section closely examines a few common pet illnesses and their successful treatments.

Among the most common health problems in pets are digestive disorders, which frequently show up as symptoms like vomiting, diarrhea, and constipation. Numerous things, such as infections, gastrointestinal diseases, food allergies, and careless eating, might contribute to these problems. Probiotics, anti-diarrheal drugs, dietary changes, and supportive care such as electrolyte and hydration supplements can all be used to treat digestive issues.

Pets frequently experience skin issues, manifesting as anything from hair loss, blemishes, and infections to itching, redness, and inflammation. Allergies, parasites, bacterial or fungal infections, hormone imbalances, or underlying medical disorders can all lead to skin problems. Topical drugs, medicated shampoos, dietary adjustments, vitamins, and treating any underlying health issues can all be used as treatments for skin problems.

Pets also frequently have respiratory infections, especially in homes with several animals or places with inadequate ventilation. Symptoms of respiratory infections might include nasal discharge, coughing, sneezing, and trouble breathing. Environmental factors like smoking or allergies, bacteria, fungi, and viruses can all lead to these diseases. Antibiotics, antiviral drugs, supportive care (using humidifiers or nebulizers), and treating any underlying medical conditions are some of the treatments for respiratory infections.

Senior pets and those with underlying orthopedic diseases like arthritis, hip dysplasia, or ligament injuries frequently have joint pain and movement problems. Limping, stiffness, resistance to movement, and trouble getting up or down stairs are possible symptoms. Some treatments for joint discomfort include physical therapy, weight control, anti-inflammatory pharmaceuticals, joint supplements like glucosamine and chondroitin, pain management medications, and lifestyle changes to lessen joint stress.

Pets with lengthy ears or floppy ear flaps that trap moisture and dirt are more susceptible to ear infections. Head shaking, scratching at the ears, foul odor, discharge, and redness or swelling of the ear canal can indicate an ear infection. Bacteria, yeast, parasites, or underlying medical disorders, including allergies or hormone imbalances, can all cause these diseases. Oral antibiotics or antifungals, topical treatments, ear cleaning, and treating any underlying medical conditions can all be part of the treatment for ear infections.

Typical pet illnesses include respiratory infections, joint pain, ear infections, and skin and digestive disorders. Comprehending the origins and manifestations of various ailments is crucial for prompt diagnosis and efficacious therapy. For pets to remain healthy and have a good quality of life, it is essential to swiftly and effectively address their health concerns related to nutrition, drugs, supplements, or supportive care. Developing a customized treatment plan that meets each pet's unique needs and promotes healing and wellness requires speaking with a licensed veterinarian.

Guidelines for safe use

Guidelines for safe use are essential yet sometimes overlooked when it comes to the responsible and successful use of herbal treatments. Even though herbs can provide several health benefits, it is necessary to approach the usage of herbs with caution and attention to achieve the best possible outcomes and reduce the likelihood of experiencing any adverse effects. It is essential to follow these principles to ensure that herbal medicine is safe and effective, regardless of whether you use herbs for yourself, your family, or an animal companion.

It is of the utmost importance to educate yourself on the herbs you intend to take, including their characteristics, the potential advantages they may offer, and any known hazards or contraindications associated with their usage. Some plants are not appropriate for everyone; in addition, certain herbs may interact with drugs or worsen certain health conditions. Spend some time conducting in-depth research on each herb and get information from respectable sources such as herbal literature, journals that have been peer-reviewed, or qualified medical professionals. This will ensure that the information you obtain is accurate and trustworthy.

In addition, it is essential to obtain herbs of superior quality from companies with a solid reputation to guarantee their safety and effectiveness. Choose herbs that have been gathered and processed responsibly, without the use of pesticides, herbicides, or any other dangerous chemicals. Look for herbs that have been wildcrafted or organically grown. Avoid purchasing herbs from unknown or questionable sources since there is a possibility that they have been adulterated or contaminated with ingredients that could be hazardous to your health.

In addition, when utilizing herbal treatments, it is essential to adhere to the appropriate dosage requirements to prevent either accidental overdose or accidental underdose. The dosage of herbs can change depending on several factors, including age, weight, current health situation, and the form and preparation of the herb. To begin with, modest doses should be taken and progressively raised as required while constantly monitoring for any adverse effects that may occur. Measurement tools such as droppers, syringes, or spoons should be used to ensure proper dosing. This is especially important when providing herbs to youngsters or animals.

In addition, it is essential to be aware of any potential adverse effects or interactions related to the herbs you are utilizing. Even while herbs are generally believed to be safe when used in the recommended manner, there are some instances in which they can induce adverse effects or interact with specific drugs. It is possible for herbs to cause a variety of adverse effects, including gastrointestinal distress, allergic responses, sleepiness, and headaches. There is also the possibility that certain herbs could interact with drugs like blood thinners, anticoagulants, or immunosuppressants, which could potentially affect the effectiveness or safety of these medications. Before using herbs, you should always get the advice of a trained medical professional, mainly if you are pregnant, breastfeeding, or taking any drugs.

In addition, it is vital to keep herbs appropriately to preserve their effectiveness and maintain their freshness over time. To prevent oxidation and degradation, herbs should be stored in an excellent, dry location shielded from direct sunlight, dampness, and heat. Additionally, herbs should be kept in airtight containers that are well-sealed. It is possible to extend the shelf life of herbs and ensure that they are effective when used if stored correctly.

To summarize, it is vital to adhere to rules for safe use when it comes to utilizing herbal treatments to promote health and well-being. Several crucial procedures must be taken to guarantee herbal medicine's safety and effectiveness. These include educating oneself about herbs, obtaining high-quality ingredients, adhering to the appropriate dosage guidelines, being aware of potential side effects and interactions, and storing herbs appropriately. By approaching the use of herbs with caution and attention, you may take advantage of their medicinal benefits while limiting the danger of harm to yourself, your family, and your pets.

CHAPTER IX

Troubleshooting and Overcoming Challenges

Common Problems and Solutions

In daily life, common difficulties will inevitably arise; the trick is to figure out how to solve them. To navigate through life with resilience and success, one must be able to recognize typical difficulties and their suitable remedies, whether they are personal or professional.

Many individuals encounter stress and overload frequently. In today's fast-paced society, it's simple to feel overburdened by the pressures of job, family, and other commitments. Establishing healthy coping strategies and emphasizing self-care to manage stress is critical to solving this issue effectively. This could entail choosing hobbies that make you happy and fulfilled, setting boundaries and refusing overly demanding obligations, practicing relaxation techniques like deep breathing, meditation, or yoga, and getting assistance from friends, family, or a therapist.

Lack of motivation and procrastination are two more prevalent issues. Many people suffer from procrastination, delaying work until the very last minute, and experiencing stress due to looming deadlines and commitments. Breaking things down into smaller, more manageable steps, making a realistic schedule or deadline for finishing them, removing distractions, and finding strategies to maintain motivation and attention are all crucial for overcoming procrastination. This could entail establishing clear objectives, praising yourself when you progress, and holding yourself responsible for keeping your course.

Furthermore, interpersonal disputes and misunderstandings are frequent problems in interactions with friends, family, coworkers, or romantic partners. To overcome these problems, it's critical to engage in effective communication, actively listen to others' viewpoints, and make an effort to comprehend their wants and feelings. This could entail having direct and honest discussions, politely and assertively expressing one's opinions and feelings, and coming up with solutions or compromises that satisfy the interests of all parties.

Financial difficulty is another prevalent issue that many people encounter at some point in their lives. Financial stress can hurt general well-being, from managing debt, worrying about the future, or having difficulty making ends meet. To deal with financial difficulties, it's critical to create and follow a budget, put needs before wants, look into ways to raise money or cut costs, and, if necessary, seek the advice of financial consultants or counselors. Stability and peace of mind can also be attained by setting long-term economic objectives and preparing for emergencies.

Furthermore, health-related difficulties are prevalent issues that can affect well-being and quality of life. For general vitality and longevity, taking care of one's health is crucial, whether by managing chronic problems, dealing with illness or injury, or adopting healthier behaviors. It's critical to prioritize self-care, keep a balanced diet, get regular exercise, get adequate sleep, and seek support and medical attention when necessary to manage health issues. Having a solid support system of friends, family, and medical professionals can also be a great way to offer support and encouragement when things go tough.

In summary, everyday issues will always arise, but overcoming them and prospering in the face of hardship depends on identifying workable answers. People can develop resilience, resourcefulness, and personal growth by recognizing typical issues like stress, procrastination, interpersonal disputes, financial troubles, and health concerns and using appropriate methods and treatments to manage them. People may handle life's ups and downs with grace and resilience if they have perseverance and self-awareness and are willing to ask for help when needed.

Addressing non-responsiveness to herbs

Addressing non-responsiveness to herbs can be confusing for those looking for natural ways to support their health and well-being. Although many people find herbs safe and beneficial, there are several situations in which people may not get the intended results or benefits from using herbs as a treatment. One way to effectively manage this issue is for people to understand what causes non-responsiveness and investigate other options.

Individual differences in physiology and biochemistry could cause non-responsiveness to herbs. Similar to traditional drugs, different people react differently to plants. Several factors, including lifestyle choices, underlying medical problems, genetic predispositions, and pharmaceutical interactions, can influence herbal metabolism and utilization inside the body. Some people may need to use other formulations, greater dosages, or different herbs to obtain the intended therapeutic results.

Another thing to consider is the quality and potency of the herbs being utilized. Herbal products are not all made equal, and differences in production, sourcing, and processing might affect their effectiveness. To guarantee the safety and efficacy of herbal remedies, it is imperative to select standardized, high-quality goods from reliable vendors. Furthermore, fresh or organically cultivated herbs may contain larger amounts of medicinal chemicals than dried or processed varieties, so certain people may benefit from using them.

Moreover, an ineffective herbal remedy could result from a mishandled dosage or administration. Herbal medicines work best when applied consistently over time and in the right dosages. For herbal remedies to work best for them, people may need to modify their dosages, usage schedules, or modes of administration. Speaking with a licensed herbalist or medical professional can assist people in creating individualized treatment programs that cater to their unique requirements and preferences.

Furthermore, if a person is not responding to herbs, underlying health problems or imbalances may need to be treated. Herbs are frequently utilized to enhance the body's innate healing abilities and to foster harmony and balance. To get the best effects from herbal remedies, treating underlying medical disorders or imbalances, such as chronic inflammation, hormone imbalances, or dietary deficiencies, in addition to existing diseases, might be necessary. Herbs can be used with complementary therapies, such as diet, lifestyle changes, and stress-reduction methods, to address underlying issues and improve general health and well-being.

Sometimes, determining why a person isn't responding to herbs takes trial and error. Finding the ideal herbal combinations, doses, and delivery systems for each person's needs may take some time and effort. Over time, keeping thorough records of herb use, symptoms, and reactions can help people monitor their progress and spot trends. It's also critical to maintain an open mind and be adaptable when investigating various strategies and modifying treatment plans as necessary.

To sum up, treating non-responsiveness to herbs requires a thorough and customized strategy that considers elements like biochemistry, the quality of the herbs, dosage, delivery, underlying medical conditions, and trial and error. By collaborating with experienced herbalists or healthcare practitioners, individuals can explore alternate ways, optimize their treatment regimens, and obtain the desired therapeutic outcomes from herbal treatments. People can use the natural therapeutic properties of herbs to promote their health and well-being if they are persistent, patient, and open to trying new things.

Managing side effects

Using any medication or treatment, including herbal therapies, requires careful consideration of potential adverse effects. While herbs are typically considered harmless when used properly, some people may experience adverse effects. People using herbal treatments to improve their health and well-being can use them safely and successfully if they know how to identify and manage these adverse effects.

Digestion disturbance is a frequent adverse reaction to herbal medicines, and it can cause symptoms like nausea, bloating, gas, or diarrhea. Some herbs can irritate the digestive tract or induce gastrointestinal pain in sensitive people, particularly those with bitter or astringent qualities. Dilute strong-tasting herbs with water or other liquids, start with modest dosages and increase gradually as tolerated, and take herbs with food to minimize discomfort and manage side effects related to the digestive system. Additionally, people experiencing nausea or indigestion may find relief using digestive aids like fennel, ginger, or peppermint.

Allergy reactions are yet another possible adverse consequence of herbal treatments, especially for those who are allergic to plants or botanicals. An allergic reaction can cause redness, swelling, hives, itching, and breathing difficulties. It's critical to stop using the offending herb when allergic reactions happen. You should also contact a doctor if symptoms worsen or don't go away. People should avoid using herbs known to cause allergies or sensitivities and conduct a patch test before using any new herbs, especially those known to cause allergies.

Furthermore, several plants might worsen preexisting medical issues or interact negatively with prescription drugs. For instance, herbs like garlic, ginkgo biloba, and St. John's wort may interact with blood thinners, antidepressants, or anti-seizure medications, compromising their efficacy or safety. Before utilizing herbs, speaking with a skilled healthcare provider to handle any interactions is vital. This is especially important if you are taking medicine or have underlying health concerns. Healthcare professionals can monitor for side effects, change dosages or treatment plans as necessary, and assist in identifying any interactions.

Some people may also experience less common adverse effects, such as headaches, vertigo, sleepiness, or behavioral or mood problems, in addition to these usual ones. If these negative effects manifest, it's crucial to stop using the herb and speak with a healthcare professional for additional assessment and advice. Medical professionals can offer supportive care to reduce symptoms, suggest substitute herbs or treatments, and assist in determining the underlying cause of side effects.

In summary, controlling side effects is crucial to safely and efficiently using herbal treatments. People may reduce the possibility of suffering unfavorable consequences from herbal remedies by being aware of potential side effects, starting with low doses, gradually increasing as tolerated, and keeping an eye out for detrimental reactions. To further assure the safety and efficacy of herbs, speak with a licensed healthcare professional before using them, particularly if you have underlying medical issues, allergies, or are on medication. People can naturally promote their health and well-being by using herbs' healing potential if they are adequately educated, aware of them, and guided in their use.

Building a Support System

Creating a support network is crucial to preserving general health and facing obstacles with courage and resiliency. A support system comprises people, places, and networks that offer social, practical, and emotional assistance when needed. A solid support network can significantly impact an individual's capacity to manage, adjust, and prosper when confronted with personal hardships, health concerns, professional obstacles, or life transitions.

Cultivating meaningful relationships with friends, family, and loved ones who provide unconditional love, encouragement, and understanding is one of the most crucial parts of creating a support system. These people offer emotional support by being a source of strength and assurance during trying times, listening intently, and sharing wise or consoling words. Building a solid support network and fostering these connections requires prioritizing quality time spent together, keeping lines of communication open and honest, and expressing gratitude for their assistance.

Getting professional assistance from therapists, counselors, or support groups can also be very helpful for dealing with particular problems or obstacles. These experts provide tools, direction, and specialized knowledge to assist people in overcoming challenging emotions, creating coping mechanisms, and pursuing personal development and healing. Whether dealing with marital troubles, mental health concerns, or life transitions, professional help can offer a secure and accepting environment where people can explore their ideas and emotions and obtain insightful viewpoints.

Creating a support system also entails finding and using networks and resources in the community that provide help and encouragement. Local groups, nonprofits, places of worship, and online communities that offer connections, resources, and information about particular needs or interests are examples of this. Whether someone needs help with money, childcare, housing support, or career advice, these community resources can help them get the tools and support they need to overcome challenges and accomplish their objectives.

Moreover, self-care activities like mindfulness, meditation, exercise, and hobbies can also be extremely important in creating a support network by fostering mental, emotional, and physical well-being. By allowing people to reflect on themselves, reduce stress, and find personal fulfillment, these activities support resilience and coping mechanisms in the face of adversity.

Maintaining a healthy lifestyle, putting rest, food, and sleep first, and looking for fulfilling and joyful pursuits are other ways to support resilience and general well- being.

To sum up, creating a support network is critical to preserving social, practical, and emotional assistance during life's ups and downs. People may build a solid and resilient support system that enables them to face life's obstacles with bravery, grit, and grace by emphasizing self-care routines, obtaining professional assistance, building meaningful relationships, and using community resources. A strong support network may be comforting, empowering, and helpful when dealing with personal troubles, health problems, job obstacles, or life changes. This, in turn, can lead to increased resilience, well-being, and life fulfillment.

Finding reliable information and support

In the current digital era, where an overwhelming amount of information is easily accessible, finding trustworthy information and support is essential. Accurate, reliable information and support networks are critical for managing life's difficulties with clarity and confidence, whether seeking help on health matters, personal challenges, or career goals.

One of the first stages in locating trustworthy information and assistance is identifying trustworthy sources and services that offer accurate, fact-based information on a particular topic. This could entail looking through reputable publications, books, articles, or journals authored by licensed experts or professionals in the topic. Seek out sites that follow ethical norms and rules for neutrality and accuracy, quote reliable research, and are upfront about the credentials and affiliations of their writers.

Additionally, while facing difficulties or looking for direction, getting assistance from competent and experienced people or organizations can offer insightful advice, encouragement, and guidance that is very helpful. Healthcare practitioners, therapists, counselors, mentors, and support groups with specialized interests or knowledge may fall under this category. These people and groups can provide individualized guidance, materials, and recommendations catered to specific requirements and situations, assisting in effectively handling issues and discovering solutions.

Building a network of dependable friends, family, and peers can offer social, practical, and emotional support when things go tough. One can develop a sense of connection, camaraderie, and belonging by surrounding themselves with people who have similar values, interests, and aspirations. This can create a supportive environment where people feel understood, accepted, and empowered. Resilience and strength can be demonstrated by individuals navigating life's problems with a solid support network, whether looking for guidance, encouragement, or just someone to listen to them.

To assess information and make decisions independently, it's crucial to develop critical thinking abilities and self-reliance, in addition to asking for help when needed. This could entail developing research, analytical, and discernment abilities to evaluate the reliability and validity of sources, challenge presumptions, and carefully consider the facts before making decisions or acting. Gaining knowledge and skills can help people become more astute information consumers and better able to negotiate the challenges of contemporary living.

Additionally, being knowledgeable about current events and pertinent topics can assist people in making wise choices and taking the initiative to solve difficulties or pursue goals effectively. Increasing knowledge and skills in particular areas of interest or competence may entail maintaining connections with reliable information sources, attending workshops or seminars, participating in online forums or discussion groups, and looking for continuing education opportunities.

In conclusion, overcoming obstacles in life and coming to wise conclusions depend on accessing trustworthy information and assistance. By identifying credible sources, consulting with knowledgeable individuals and organizations, developing supportive networks, and refining critical thinking abilities, individuals can equip themselves with the necessary knowledge, resources, and assistance to effectively address issues, surmount challenges, and accomplish their objectives. A strong foundation for success and well-being can be established by accessing reliable, accurate information and encouraging networks, whether seeking help on health matters, personal struggles, or career goals.

Joining herbal communities

Although we live in a society becoming more and more dominated by fast-paced lifestyles and quick pleasures, timeless wisdom encourages us to slow down, reconnect with nature, and embrace the healing power of herbs. Participating in herbal communities is not just about taking up a new pastime or following a fad; it is a meaningful journey of connection, learning, and development that covers our existence's physical, emotional, and spiritual aspects.

The profound appreciation that herbal communities have for the natural environment and its many benefits is at the center of their existence. Individuals engage in a journey of discovery when they become members of these societies, immersing themselves in the vast body of herbal knowledge handed down from generation to generation. Ancient wisdom and contemporary scientific research come together in this place, resulting in a synergy that promotes holistic healing and well-being. By taking part in herbal communities, individuals can access a wealth of information, including the therapeutic characteristics of particular plants and the art of producing herbal treatments.

In addition, one can have a sense of belonging and connection by participating in herbal communities, which are sometimes absent in today's fractured society. People who are passionate about plants and profoundly respect the natural world can find people who share their love and respect for the natural world in these communities. Herbal communities provide opportunities for individuals who have similar interests to interact with one another, share their thoughts, and develop meaningful connections. These possibilities can be online forums, in-person meet-ups, or workshops. Live in a world that places excessive importance on individualism rather than community. Joining herbal communities can provide you with a potent remedy: the opportunity to create relationships founded on shared ideals and a shared respect for the planet.

In addition to the practical advantages of gaining knowledge about herbs and making connections with people who share similar interests, participation in herbal communities also encourages personal development and the finding of one's own identity. The more one explores the realm of herbalism, the more likely one will come across novel concepts, points of view, and ways of being. In addition to gaining a deeper awareness of themselves and their place in the world, they may discover previously unknown abilities or passions, find new ways to express themselves or discover new avenues for personal expression. In this sense, herbal communities act as catalysts for transformation, inviting individuals to explore new paths, confront old beliefs, and embrace a higher level of authenticity in their way of life.

Herbal communities provide an excellent chance for healing, both on an individual and a communal level, and the most important benefit of joining such communities. Herbal medicine offers a mild yet effective treatment for the disorders that are associated with modern living, which are characterized by chronic stress, excessive work, and the degradation of the environment. Individuals can restore a sense of empowerment and agency in a world that can be overwhelming by learning to harness the healing power of plants. This allows them to take charge of their health and well-being, restoring their sense of agency. Furthermore, individuals can magnify the healing effects of herbs by coming together in a community, which creates a ripple effect that goes far beyond the person to embrace families, communities, and even the planet itself. This is because the healing powers of herbs are amplified when individuals come together.

In conclusion, becoming a member of herbal communities is not only about gaining knowledge or becoming proficient in a new skill; it is a profound journey of connection, learning, and development that includes every facet of our existence. By participating in herbal communities, individuals can access vast information, establish meaningful connections with others, and begin a journey of individual and community healing. Herbal communities are a ray of light in a world that frequently appears to be fractured and unconnected. They remind us of our profound interconnection with the natural world and one another. As we come together as a community and accept the knowledge that plants have to offer, we not only cure ourselves but also contribute to the earth's healing. This is a witness to the enduring ability of herbalism to alter lives and design a more sustainable and harmonious future.

CHAPTER X

Case Studies and Success Stories

Real-Life Examples

This section provides convincing evidence of the practical application and effectiveness of herbal medicine in resolving various health conditions and increasing overall well-being through real-life situations. The following instances offer invaluable insights into how individuals have included herbal treatments in their healthcare routines, frequently improving their health and quality of life. By examining these real-life situations, we can acquire a more profound comprehension of the adaptability, effectiveness, and holistic significance of herbal medicine.

A middle-aged woman who was battling with chronic migraines that had a substantial influence on her day-to-day life and overall well-being is a real-life example that is particularly moving. The traditional treatments had only provided a limited amount of relief and were accompanied by side effects that were difficult to tolerate. She was in desperate need of relief, so she sought the advice of an expert herbalist. The herbalist suggested that she take a combination of supplements containing butterbur (Petasites hybridus) and feverfew (Tanacetum parthenium), both well-known for their capacity to lessen the frequency and intensity of migraines. The woman was able to resume her typical activities and reclaim a sense of control over her health after experiencing a notable reduction in the frequency and intensity of her migraines over many months of constant use. Herbal remedies can provide safe and effective relief from chronic health disorders that may not react appropriately to conventional therapies. This real-life example demonstrates the potential of herbal medicines to offer such relief.

An additional interesting real-life case includes a small child who was afflicted with recurring ear infections that were resistant to the treatment provided by antibiotics. The mother of the child was looking for a substitute that was less harsh because she was concerned about the long-term consequences that antibiotics would have on her child's immune system and gut health. Garlic-infused olive oil drops are a traditional medicine that is known for its antibacterial and anti-inflammatory characteristics. She began using these drops in her child's ears after consulting with an experienced herbalist. Her satisfaction was brought on by the fact that the child's ear infections disappeared a few days after beginning the herbal treatment, and later ear examinations proved no infection. Herbal medicines are beneficial in treating common childhood diseases and decreasing the need for antibiotics, as demonstrated by this real-life example.

In addition, a real-life case of an older man who was battling with insomnia and other sleep problems provides insight into the therapeutic benefits of herbal medicine for the support of sleep. Even though he tried several different prescription sleep aids, the guy continued to have trouble falling asleep and staying asleep, which had a detrimental influence on his general health and quality of life. In his search for a natural alternative, he sought the advice of an herbalist, who suggested that he take a combination of valerian (Valeriana officinalis) and passionflower (Passiflora incarnata) pills. Both of these plants are well-known for their soothing and relaxing effects. The man noticed considerable changes in the quality and duration of his sleep within a few weeks of beginning the herbal regimen. As a result, he could wake up feeling revitalized and refreshed. Herbal remedies can promote restful sleep and improve general well-being without the risk of dependency or unpleasant side effects linked with prescription sleep aids. This real-life example demonstrates the potential of herbal remedies to accomplish these goals.

Herbal medication is effective in alleviating typical pregnancy-related symptoms, as demonstrated by a real-life case involving a pregnant woman who experienced nausea and vomiting during the first trimester of her pregnancy. She was looking for a natural solution to reduce her agony since she was concerned about the harmful effects that pharmaceutical anti-nausea pills could have on her unborn child. After consulting with a certified herbalist, she began consuming ginger (Zingiber officinale) tea and candies, both of which are well-known for their ability to prevent nausea. The ginger supplied significant alleviation from her symptoms, much to her surprise. As a result, she was able to take pleasure in her pregnancy to a greater extent and without the anxiety that she would cause harm to her unborn child. This real-life example demonstrates that herbal treatments are safe and helpful in promoting the health and well-being of mothers during pregnancy.

It is also possible to gain an understanding of the therapeutic benefits of herbal medicine for mental and emotional well-being by looking at a real-life scenario that involves a middle-aged guy who is battling chronic stress and anxiety. Even though he tried several different pharmaceutical treatments, the guy continued to experience symptoms, and he subsequently looked for a more holistic approach to controlling his disease. He started using adaptogenic herbs in his daily routine, such as ashwagandha (Withania somnifera), holy basil (Ocimum sanctum), and Rhodiola (Rhodiola rosea), with the assistance of a herbalist who provided him with direction. Over time, he observed a notable decrease in his levels of anxiety, an improvement in his mood, and an increase in his resilience to the effects of stressors. The function that herbal medicine plays in promoting emotional equilibrium and sustaining mental health is brought to light by this real-life example.

Furthermore, a real-life example of a person battling digestive disorders provides insight into the therapeutic benefits of herbal medicine for the health of the gastrointestinal tract. The client continued to endure discomfort, bloating, and irregular bowel movements even though they tried a variety of drugs that were available without a prescription online. When looking for a natural option, they sought the advice of a herbalist who suggested taking peppermint (Mentha piperita) and chamomile (Matricaria chamomilla) pills. Both of these herbs are well-known for their ability to calm the digestive tract and reduce inflammation. After beginning the herbal regimen, the individual noticed considerable improvements in their digestive problems within a short period. These benefits included a reduction in bloating, an improvement in regularity, and an overall improvement in comfort. Herbal medicines have the potential to alleviate common gastrointestinal symptoms and improve digestive well-being, as demonstrated by this real-life example.

In conclusion, real-life examples of herbal medicine in action prove the practical application of herbal remedies and the efficiency of these treatments in promoting healing and supporting health. Herbs provide a natural and comprehensive approach to addressing a wide range of health conditions, including alleviating symptoms connected to pregnancy, reducing stress and anxiety, improving sleep quality, relieving migraines and ear infections, and supporting digestive health. We can acquire significant insights into how herbs can be utilized to promote health, enhance vitality, and improve quality of life for individuals of all ages and walks of life by going through individual examples in which herbal medicine has been shown to have a good influence.

Detailed case studies

The practical use and efficacy of herbal medicine in resolving specific health conditions and increasing overall well-being are examined in more detail through detailed case studies, which offer deep and nuanced insights into the subject matter. By examining real-life examples in which individuals have utilized herbal remedies as part of their healthcare regimen, we can acquire a more profound comprehension of the complexity of herbal medicine and its ability to enhance healing and vitality.

A woman in her middle years who suffered from persistent headaches that had a significant negative influence on her quality of life is the subject of an intriguing case study situation. Only a tiny amount of alleviation had been supplied by traditional treatments, which were also accompanied by unwelcome side effects. In her search for a natural option, she sought the advice of an expert herbalist, who suggested that she take a combination of supplements containing butterbur (Petasites hybridus) and feverfew (Tanacetum parthenium). These herbs are well-known for their capacity to lessen the frequency and intensity of migraines. The woman was able to resume her typical activities and reclaim a sense of control over her health after experiencing a considerable reduction in the frequency and intensity of her migraines over many months of constant use. Herbal remedies can provide safe and effective relief from chronic health disorders that may not react satisfactorily to conventional treatments. This example demonstrates the potential of herbal medicines to perform this function.

A little boy suffering from recurring ear infections resistant to antibiotic treatment is the subject of yet another exciting case study. The mother of the child was looking for a substitute that was less harsh because she was concerned about the long-term consequences that antibiotics would have on her child's immune system and gut health. Garlic-infused olive oil drops are a traditional medicine that is known for its antibacterial and anti-inflammatory characteristics. She began using these drops in her child's ears after consulting with an experienced herbalist. Her satisfaction was brought on by the fact that the child's ear infections disappeared a few days after beginning the herbal treatment, and later ear examinations proved no infection. The usefulness of herbal therapies in treating common childhood diseases and decreasing the need for antibiotics is demonstrated by this particular case study.

In addition, a comprehensive case study that focuses on an older man who is battling with insomnia and other sleep problems provides significant insight into the therapeutic benefits of herbal medication to provide support for sleep. Even though he tried several different prescription sleep aids, the guy continued to have trouble falling asleep and staying asleep, which had a detrimental influence on his general health and quality of life. In his search for a natural alternative, he sought the advice of an herbalist, who suggested that he take a combination of valerian (Valeriana officinalis) and passionflower (Passiflora incarnata) pills. Both of these plants are well-known for their soothing and relaxing effects. The man noticed considerable changes in the quality and duration of his sleep within a few weeks of beginning the herbal regimen. As a result, he could wake up feeling revitalized and refreshed. Herbal treatments can promote undisturbed sleep and improve general well-being without the risk of dependency or unpleasant side effects linked with prescription sleep aids. This case demonstrates the potential of herbal remedies to accomplish these goals.

In addition, a comprehensive case study that describes the experience of a pregnant woman who was experiencing nausea and vomiting during the first trimester of her pregnancy provides valuable insight into the effectiveness of herbal medication in alleviating common symptoms associated with pregnancy. She was looking for a natural solution to reduce her agony since she was concerned about the harmful effects that pharmaceutical anti-nausea pills could have on her unborn child. After consulting with a certified herbalist, she began consuming ginger (Zingiber officinale) tea and candies, both of which are well-known for their ability to prevent nausea. The ginger supplied significant alleviation from her symptoms, much to her surprise. As a result, she was able to take pleasure in her pregnancy to a greater extent and without the anxiety that she would cause harm to her unborn child. The findings of this case demonstrate that herbal treatments are both safe and beneficial in promoting maternal health and well-being throughout pregnancy.

In addition, a comprehensive case study that focuses on a middle-aged man who is battling with chronic stress and anxiety to provide insight into the therapeutic effects of herbal medicine for mental and emotional well-being is presented. Even though he tried several different pharmaceutical treatments, the guy continued to experience symptoms, and he subsequently looked for a more holistic approach to controlling his disease. He started using adaptogenic herbs in his daily routine, such as ashwagandha (Withania somnifera), holy basil (Ocimum sanctum), and Rhodiola (Rhodiola rosea), with the assistance of a herbalist who provided him with direction. Over time, he observed a notable decrease in his levels of anxiety, an improvement in his mood, and an increase in his resilience to the effects of stressors. This particular instance sheds light on the positive impact that herbal medicine can have on mental health and the maintenance of emotional equilibrium.

Additional information regarding the therapeutic benefits of herbal medicine for gastrointestinal health can be gleaned from a comprehensive case study that focuses on an individual experiencing digestive system difficulties. The client continued to endure discomfort, bloating, and irregular bowel movements even though they tried a variety of drugs that were available without a prescription online. When looking for a natural option, they sought the advice of a herbalist who suggested taking peppermint (Mentha piperita) and chamomile (Matricaria chamomilla) pills. Both of these herbs are well-known for their ability to calm the digestive tract and reduce inflammation. After beginning the herbal regimen, the individual noticed considerable improvements in their digestive problems within a short period. These benefits included a reduction in bloating, an improvement in regularity, and an overall improvement in comfort. In light of this situation, it is clear that herbal medicines have the potential to alleviate common gastrointestinal symptoms and improve digestive well-being.

When addressing various health issues, thorough case studies provide significant insights into the practical application of herbal medicine and its success. Herbs offer a natural and comprehensive approach to health and healing, from the relief of migraines and ear infections to the improvement of sleep quality, the alleviation of symptoms connected to pregnancy, the reduction of stress and anxiety, and the support of digestive health. By examining specific instances in which herbal medicine has been shown to have a beneficial effect, we can get a more profound appreciation for the adaptability, effectiveness, and holistic character of herbal medicines from the perspective of health promotion.

Key takeaways and insights

Regarding the holistic approach to health and well-being, the major takeaways and insights that can be gained from the study of herbal medicine offer profound teachings and views. Through investigation and analysis, several central themes emerge, each offering valuable insights into herbs' potential to support health, facilitate healing, and enhance quality of life.

When it comes to attaining optimal health, one of the most essential things that can be learned from the study of herbal medicine is the identification of the interconnectedness of the body, mind, and spirit. Herbalism recognizes that mental, emotional, and spiritual well-being are intricately connected with physical health, and it emphasizes treating the whole person rather than merely treating the symptoms of a specific illness through medicine. Herbal medicine is an approach to health care that is both comprehensive and holistic. It tries to restore balance and promote well-being on various levels by addressing imbalances and disharmonies at all levels because it addresses these issues.

Furthermore, the study of herbal medicine shines a light on the significance of tailored and personalized care in health and healing. Herbalists must acknowledge that everyone is different and may react differently to herbs and other therapeutic means. Herbalists can create treatment programs to match each individual's specific requirements and objectives by considering aspects such as the individual's constitution, lifestyle, and personal preferences. This individualized method of providing medical care ensures that therapy is successful and empowering. This is because individuals are actively involved in their healing process and are given the ability to make educated decisions regarding their health.

Recognizing nature's underlying wisdom and healing power is yet another significant insight that can be learned through the study of herbal medicine. To take advantage of herbs' medicinal and therapeutic benefits, cultures worldwide have been using them for millennia. Herbalists have identified and produced many plants with specific actions and properties to support your health and promote healing. This has been accomplished through careful observation, experimentation, and tradition. Herbal medicine is a method of providing health care that is both natural and sustainable, and it follows the natural rhythms and cycles of the natural world. It does this by harnessing the healing power of nature.

Further, the study of herbal medicine highlights the significance of preventative measures and proactive self-care in preserving health and well-being. The practice of herbal medicine argues for adopting preventative measures to maintain health and prevent imbalances before they develop instead of waiting until illness or disease has already manifested. To achieve this, it may be necessary to embrace good lifestyle habits such as proper eating, regular exercise, stress management, and adequate rest, as well as to incorporate herbs and other natural medicines into daily routines to enhance resilience and vitality. Herbal medicine allows people to take charge of their health and improve their well-being by emphasizing the importance of preventative measures and proactive self-care.

In addition, the study of herbal medicine brings to light the significance of joint efforts and integration in medical care. Herbalism is not a stand-alone practice; instead, it is a medical and therapeutic approach that works in conjunction with and compliments other styles of treatment. In providing holistic and all-encompassing care to their patients, herbalists frequently collaborate with other medical professionals, such as medical doctors, naturopathic physicians, and complementary therapists, to give holistic and thorough care. To provide more effective and integrated care that caters to the many requirements of individuals and communities, healthcare practitioners must first acknowledge the benefits and drawbacks of various therapeutic approaches and then collaborate in an atmosphere of collaboration and mutual respect.

In conclusion, the study of herbal medicine provides essential insights and critical takeaways that can contribute to our comprehension of health, healing, and overall well-being. By recognizing the interconnectedness of the body, mind, and spirit, harnessing the healing power of nature, embracing individualized and personalized care, promoting prevention and proactive self-care, and fostering collaboration and integration in health care, herbal medicine offers a holistic and comprehensive approach to health that honors the innate wisdom of the body and supports the inherent capacity for healing and vitality. Herbal medicine includes all of these aspects. We may build a more profound connection, balance, and well-being for ourselves, our communities, and our planet as we continue to investigate and incorporate the principles and practices of herbal medicine into our lives and healthcare systems. This will allow us to fulfill our potential better.

CONCLUSION

Conclusively, "Natural Infection Fighters - Effective Herbal Antibiotics for Everyday Use" provides a thorough and perceptive examination of the potential of herbal medicine to promote health and combat illnesses. Within the pages of this electronic book, readers have encountered abundant knowledge regarding different herbs, their characteristics, applications, preparations, and usefulness in treating common illnesses and enhancing general health. This e-book is an invaluable tool for anybody interested in utilizing nature's healing power, covering topics such as immunity and infections and the methods, dosage, safety measures, and applications of herbal antibiotics for specific health issues.

Through an exploration of authentic scenarios and comprehensive case studies, readers have acquired a pragmatic understanding regarding the efficaciousness of herbal remedies in managing an extensive array of health concerns, encompassing migraines, ear infections, sleep disruptions, symptoms associated with pregnancy, stress, anxiety, and digestive disorders. These true stories demonstrate herbal therapy's adaptability, effectiveness, and all-encompassing qualities in fostering well-being and recovery on various levels.

Furthermore, the study of herbal medicine has yielded important insights and takeaways highlighting the value of proactive self-care, prevention, teamwork, and integration in healthcare. By realizing the interconnectedness of body, mind, and spirit and using the healing power of nature, people can take proactive measures to support their health and well-being and build a greater sense of connection, balance, and energy in their lives.

All things considered, "Natural Infection Fighters— Effective Herbal Antibiotics for Everyday Use" gives readers the tools they need to take charge of their health and consider natural remedies instead of artificial ones. The knowledge and perspectives offered in this e- book will direct you to maximum health and vitality via herbal medicine, whether your goals are to strengthen your immune system, reduce the symptoms of common illnesses, or improve your general well-being.

Thank you for buying and reading/listening to our book. If you found this book useful/helpful please take a few minutes and leave a review on the platform where you purchased our book. Your feedback matters greatly to us.

Printed in Great Britain
by Amazon